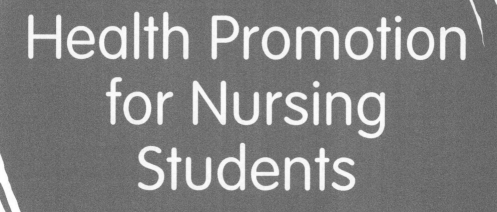

Health Promotion for Nursing Students

2E

Paul Linsley
Coralie Roll

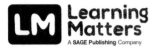

Learning Matters
A SAGE Publishing Company
1 Oliver's Yard
55 City Road
London EC1Y 1SP

SAGE Publications Inc.
2455 Teller Road
Thousand Oaks, California 91320

SAGE Publications India Pvt Ltd
B 1/I 1 Mohan Co-operative Industrial
Area
Mathura Road
New Delhi 110 044

SAGE Publications Asia-Pacific Pte Ltd
3 Church Street
#10-04 Samsung Hub
Singapore 049483

Editor: Martha Cunneen
Development editor: Eleanor Rivers
Senior project editor: Chris Marke
Project management: River Editorial
Marketing manager: Ruslana Khatagova
Cover design: Sheila Tong
Typeset by: C&M Digitals (P) Ltd, Chennai, India
Printed in the UK

Library of Congress Control Number: 2022948451

British Library Cataloguing in Publication data

A catalogue record for this book is available from
the British Library

ISBN 978-1-5297-9389-5
ISBN 978-1-5297-9388-8 (pbk)

At SAGE we take sustainability seriously. Most of our products are printed in the UK using responsibly sourced
papers and boards. When we print overseas we ensure that sustainable papers are used as measured by the
PREPS grading system. We undertake an annual audit to monitor our sustainability.

Contents

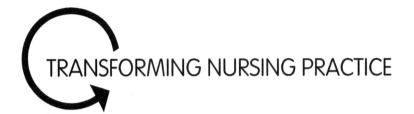

TRANSFORMING NURSING PRACTICE

Transforming Nursing Practice is a series tailor made for pre-registration student nurses. Each book in the series is:

✓ Affordable

✓ Full of active learning features

✓ Mapped to the NMC Standards of proficiency for registered nurses

✓ Focused on applying theory to practice

Each book addresses a core topic and has been carefully developed to be simple to use, quick to read and written in clear language.

An invaluable series of books that explicitly relates to the NMC standards. Each book covers a different topic that students need to explore in order to develop into a qualified nurse... I would recommend this series to all Pre-Registered nursing students whatever their field or year of study.

LINDA ROBSON,
Senior Lecturer at Edge Hill University

Many titles in the series are on our recommended reading list and for good reason - the content is up to date and easy to read. These are the books that actually get used beyond training and into your nursing career.

EMMA LYDON,
Adult Student Nursing

ABOUT THE SERIES EDITORS

DR MOOI STANDING is an Independent Nursing Consultant (UK and International) and is responsible for the core knowledge, adult nursing and personal and professional learning skills titles. She is an experienced NMC Quality Assurance Reviewer of educational programmes and a Professional Regulator Panellist on the NMC Practice Committee. Mooi is also Board member of Special Olympics Malaysia, enabling people with intellectual disabilities to participate in sports and athletics nationally and internationally.

DR SANDRA WALKER is a Clinical Academic in Mental Health working between Southern Health Trust and the University of Southampton and responsible for the mental health nursing titles. She is a Qualified Mental Health Nurse with a wide range of clinical experience spanning more than 25 years.

BESTSELLING TEXTBOOKS

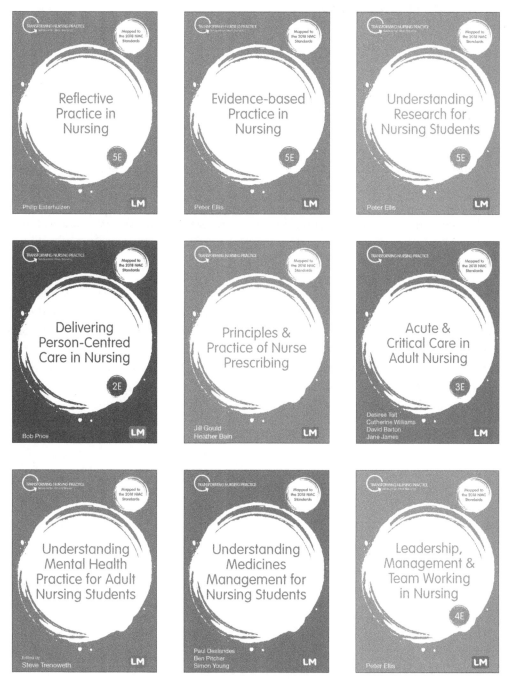

You can find a full list of textbooks in the *Transforming Nursing Practice* series at

https://uk.sagepub.com/TNP-series

About the authors

Paul Linsley is an associate professor for the University of East Anglia (UEA). He teaches on a number of courses, both single and joint honours undergraduate programmes, research master's programmes, and pre- and post-registration specialist programmes. He supervises doctoral students and sits on a number of interest panels and committees. Paul has worked on a number of research projects both as part of a team and as principal investigator. Paul has presented at international conferences and holds a number of awards. He is the author of several textbooks on nursing and health-related matters, one of which has been translated into Arabic and another into Japanese. Paul has an interest in values-based practice, and this is reflected in his work both as a clinician and as an academic.

Coralie Roll is an associate professor of nursing sciences at the University of East Anglia (UEA) and the professional lead for Pre-Registration Nursing. She had a varied clinical career as a registered adult nurse and a registered midwife before qualifying and working for several years as a specialist community public health nurse (school nursing). In 2014, Coralie gained an MSc in Clinical Research and began working as a lecturer in the UEA School of Health Sciences, where she teaches students from all fields of nursing and works with colleagues from education, health and research. Her specialist area is health promotion and public health.

For Andrew, Nathan and George (CR)

Introduction

Who is this book for?

The book explores health promotion in nursing practice. It is an introductory text to increase your awareness of the health and well-being needs of people, families and carers, communities and populations. The book will enable you to explore various aspects involved with the promotion of health and well-being in a wide range of contexts. It has been specifically written to support student nurses from all fields of nursing in developing their knowledge and skills throughout their studies. However, the book is equally helpful to all healthcare students and professionals who are working in a variety of healthcare contexts. The book acknowledges the impact that COVID-19 has had on individual and population health and on health promotion as a topic of interest and this is reflected in each of the 12 chapters.

Book structure

The 12 chapters of this book explore the following elements:

Chapter 1: Health promotion theory

This chapter looks at the thinking underpinning health promotion and some of its main components. In particular, it looks at the theory and models underpinning health promotion interventions. The chapter acts as an introduction to the topic and sets the scene for the rest of the book.

Chapter 2: Core skills for health promotion

This chapter looks at the fundamental skills required of the nurse to successfully deliver health promotion activities when working with individuals and their families. It starts by outlining the skills required of the nurse before exploring each in greater detail. It then looks at how these skills might be employed in clinical practice. The chapter enables you to explore the challenges and barriers faced by nurses providing public health interventions, as well as the many ways in which the nurse can promote and help protect good health and well-being through the nurse–patient relationship.

Chapter 3: Making every contact count (MECC)

This chapter builds on the skills introduced in Chapter 2 and focuses on a health promotion intervention that nurses are obligated to pursue in clinical practice. Making every contact count is an approach that utilises the millions of day-to-day interactions that organisations and people have with other people to encourage changes in behaviour that have a positive effect on the health and well-being of individuals, communities and populations. Central to this approach is the need to actively engage and seek out opportunities to promote health where and when they present.

Chapter 4: Health promotion with individuals

This chapter introduces you to the various elements we can consider when working with people to improve their health and well-being, including consideration of social ecological factors. Health promoting activities are important to not only enable people to live well for longer, but also take control to manage their own health and well-being. Central to this approach is the importance of the person being empowered to actively engage in their own health management.

Chapter 5: Health promotion and the family

This chapter focuses on the importance of families within health promotion. It will clarify what health education is and consider the importance of health literacy to effective health education activities. We will take a life course perspective to explore the influence of families on the health and well-being of their family members, as well as considering factors that influence effective coping and resilience within families.

Chapter 6: Health promotion at a community level

This chapter enables you to develop an appreciation of how community empowerment can support sustainable provision of services at a time when there are significant pressures on resources. We explore the various types of communities, as well as how marginalisation can adversely affect people's health and well-being. We consider asset-based approaches to community engagement, as well as how people can be engaged within communities to improve health and well-being. Finally, we discuss how nurses and multi-agency colleagues can work with people and communities to support innovative and sustainable service delivery.

Chapter 7: Health promotion at a population level

This chapter explores the promotion of health and well-being at the population level. We consider the role of public health departments, as well as how health surveillance shapes our understanding of the needs of the population to enable national and local government to set key population health strategic objectives. You will explore health surveillance data in order to highlight the importance of developing your awareness of this evidence and its use within your practice. Finally, we consider how population health targets are addressed through a multifaceted approach, which includes developing strategic policies, implementation of regulation and health promotion campaigns.

Chapter 8: Promoting health in diverse and vulnerable populations

This chapter looks at health promotion needs and approaches of emerging populations, diverse communities and vulnerable peoples. Chances for good health are not equally distributed in our societies, which causes health inequities. There is mounting evidence that some processes and conditions systematically prohibit or restrict population groups from gaining economic, social, political and cultural inclusion, and these factors are strongly associated with inequities in health status and access to health services. These factors are explored as part of this chapter, as is the role of health services and nurses in promoting health in diverse and vulnerable groups of people.

Chapter 9: Health promotion and emergent technologies

This chapter looks at emergent technologies and health promotion. The term 'emergent technologies' commonly refers to technologies that are currently developing or that are expected to be available within the next five to ten years, and is usually reserved for technologies that are creating, or are expected to create, significant social or economic effects. A range of digitised health promotion practices have emerged in the digital era. Some of these practices are voluntarily undertaken by people who are interested in improving their health and fitness, but many others are employed in the interests of organisations and agencies. This chapter looks at the use of emergent technologies, particularly digital applications and their use in health promotion.

Chapter 10: Evaluating health promotion

This chapter is designed to get you thinking about the topic under investigation and how you might go about approaching an evaluation in clinical practice as part of a health promotion intervention. It starts by exploring what we mean by 'evaluation' and why we might choose to undertake an evaluation of a health promotion intervention. The main body of the chapter looks at the role of the nurse in supporting evaluation initiatives and the process of conducting them, as well as looking at the types of evaluation available to clinical practice.

Chapter 11: Promoting one's own health

This chapter looks at how we might go about promoting our own health needs. In looking to promote the good health of others, we should not forget ourselves. A resilient, healthy nursing workforce is vital for health services and our own well-being. The chapter looks at a number of ways to think about your own health and well-being. Looking after yourself and having mechanisms in place to cope with the stress and demands of nursing practice will help to protect your health and contribute to the health and well-being of those you look after and care for.

Chapter 12: Future trends: challenges and opportunities in health promotion

This final chapter explores future trends in relation to health promotion. This includes the influence of globalisation, as well as how the political landscape can influence population and global policies that impact on health and well-being. We briefly consider healthcare developments that impact on people across the lifespan before focusing on current and future implications of changes to health service delivery.

Requirements for Future Nurse: Standards of Proficiency for Registered Nurses

Each chapter of this book begins by identifying the related platforms and proficiencies from *Future Nurse: Standards of Proficiency for Registered Nurses* (NMC, 2018a).

The Nursing and Midwifery Council (NMC) established these standards of proficiency to meet the dynamic nature of nursing in contemporary healthcare provision. All pre-registration nursing students will need to meet these proficiencies to be able to register as a nurse on completion of their studies. The proficiencies specify the expected knowledge, skills, values and behaviours of the future nurse, and are organised across seven 'platforms'. These are: (1) being an accountable professional; (2) promoting health and preventing ill health; (3) assessing needs and planning care; (4) providing and evaluating care; (5) leading and managing nursing care and working in teams; (6) improving safety and quality of care; and (7) co-ordinating care.

The standards apply across all four fields of nursing (adult, children, learning disability and mental health).

Learning features

Learning from reading text is not always easy. Therefore, to provide variety and to assist with the development of independent learning skills and the application of theory to practice, this book contains activities, case studies, scenarios, further reading, useful websites and other materials to enable you to participate in your own learning. You will need to develop your own study skills and 'learn how to learn' to get the best from the material. The book cannot provide all the answers, but instead provides a framework for your learning.

In particular, the activities in the book will help you to make sense of, and learn about, the material being presented. Some activities ask you to reflect on aspects of practice, or your experience of it, or the people or situations you encounter. *Reflection* is an essential skill in nursing, and it helps you to understand the world around you and often to identify how things might be improved. Other activities will help you develop key graduate skills, such as your ability to *think critically* about a topic in order to challenge received wisdom, or your ability to *research a topic and find appropriate information and evidence*, and to be able to *make decisions* using that evidence in situations that are often difficult and time pressured. Communication and working as part of a team are core to all nursing practice, and some activities will ask you to carry out *teamwork activities* or think about your *communication skills* to help develop these. Finally, as a registered nurse, you will be expected to *lead and manage* your own team, caseload or area of care, and so some activities focus on helping you to build confidence in doing this.

All the activities require you to take a break from reading the text, think through the issues presented and carry out some independent study, possibly using the internet. Where appropriate, there are brief outline answers presented at the end of each chapter, and these will help you to understand more fully your own reflections and independent study. Remember, academic study will always require independent work; attending lectures will never be enough to be successful on your programme, and these activities will help to deepen your knowledge and understanding of the issues under scrutiny, as well as giving you practice at working on your own.

You might want to think about completing these activities as part of your personal development plan (PDP) or portfolio. After completing an activity, write it up in your PDP or portfolio in a section devoted to that particular proficiency, then look back over time to see how far you have developed. You can also do more of the activities for a proficiency in which you have identified a weakness, which will help to build your skill and confidence in this area.

This book also contains a glossary on page 195 to assist you with unfamiliar terms. Glossary terms are in bold in the first instance that they appear.

We hope that you will find this book interesting and enjoy developing your knowledge to support your nursing practice.

Chapter 1 · Health promotion theory

Chapter aims

After reading this chapter, you will be able to:

- define the terms 'health' and 'health promotion';
- explain and describe the nurse's role in promoting health and well-being;
- understand and integrate theories and models of health promotion into nursing practice.

Introduction

This chapter introduces health promotion and its key components. It starts by looking at what it is to be healthy. It then looks at the origins of health promotion and how the concept has developed over time. The nurse's role in delivering health promotion initiatives is explored and the importance of integrated care is emphasised. The chapter then goes on to look at some of the more popular health promotion theories and models to help you start thinking about your health promotion practice. The chapter ends with a summary of the main points and suggestions for further reading.

What is health? What is it to be healthy?

Before we can look at health promotion, we need to be clear what we mean by the term 'health', the thing we are looking to promote. In order to start to do this, read the following case study.

Case study: Dorothy

Dorothy is in good health for her age of 64. She takes regular exercise and walks two to three miles per day. She pursues a balanced diet and is careful to watch her weight. Dorothy enjoys socialising and takes several holidays a year with her husband in their caravan. Dorothy has always avoided tobacco and drank alcohol in moderation and generally looks after her well-being. At a recent health check with her general practitioner (GP), Dorothy's blood pressure was a little elevated for someone of her age, with a reading of 140/90 at rest. While the GP reassured Dorothy that there was no cause for alarm, Dorothy is to monitor her blood pressure with the help of the practice nurse. Normal blood pressure is not always easy to maintain as our genetic make-up and everyday stressors can make it fluctuate. Dorothy considers herself to be healthy despite the reading, and the nurse encourages her to continue to keep fit, eat well and exercise regularly and avoid unnecessary stress. There are many reasons why Dorothy's blood pressure may have been elevated on the day of her visit to her GP and it is important to work with Dorothy to understand this and to maintain a healthy lifestyle.

Health can be defined as physical, mental and social well-being, as well as a resource for living a full life:

- Physical health covers such things as the ability to mobilise, take fluids and complete physical tasks. Physical well-being involves pursuing a healthy lifestyle to decrease the risk of disease and injury while maintaining physical fitness.

- Social health includes the ability to socialise and function as part of a group and use public services, as well as to be liked and accepted. The way that you connect to people around you, adapt to different social situations and experience a sense of belonging all contribute to your social health and well-being.
- Mental health refers to a person's emotional, social and psychological well-being. Good mental health includes the ability to control and manage emotions, concentrate on what you are doing, use memory and express emotion.

Think of these three elements as being interlinked and dependent on one another. For example, if you are feeling low in mood (mental health), you may neglect your personal hygiene (physical health) and not want to mix or socialise with others (social health). It is important to approach health as a whole rather than its different types. Good health is when all three are working together to create a feeling of well-being. Dorothy can be said to be well, as she is able to meet her physical needs, is happy socialising, and is enjoying life.

Health promotion

Health promotion has been defined by the World Health Organization (WHO) as *the process of enabling people to increase control over, and to improve their health* (WHO, 1985, page 5). It is concerned not only with treating illness and disease, but helping people achieve optimum health and well-being despite the presence of a long-term condition and maintaining a level of good health for as long as is possible. Furthermore, health promotion is a process directed towards enabling people to take responsibility and take charge of their own health and well-being. It is not something that is done on or to people; it is done by, with and for people either as individuals or as groups.

Health promotion focuses on **holistically** addressing health issues, as opposed to lecturing individuals concerning habits that are negatively affecting their health. Often individuals are aware of health practices they should adopt (e.g. exercise) or stop (e.g. smoking), but for whatever reason are unable to do so.

The fundamental aim of health promotion is to empower an individual or a community to take control of aspects of their lives that have a detrimental effect on their health, as well as for individuals to take on a healthier **lifestyle**. Health promotion is the process of enabling people to increase control over, and to improve, their health. This is a departure from the more traditional medical model of healthcare of addressing the symptoms rather than the causes of ill health and has resulted in a number of changes to the role of the nurse, as well as the way in which they practise.

The origin of health promotion

The term 'health promotion' was coined by the medical historian Henry E. Sigerist in 1945, who defined the four major tasks of medicine as: (1) promotion of health;

(2) prevention of illness; (3) restoration of the sick; and (4) active rehabilitation. He suggested that health was promoted by providing a decent standard of living, good working conditions, education, rest and recreation. This, he went on to say, required the co-ordinated efforts of political leaders, labour, industry, educators and physicians. Sigerist's (1941) observation that *promotion of health obviously tends to prevent illness, yet effective prevention calls for special measures* (page 93) illustrates the complexity of health promotion. Some diseases, such as those we are born with or inherit through our genes, cannot currently be prevented. On the other hand, many other causes of ill health are preventable with targeted intervention, such as immunisation programmes aimed at specific diseases. However, we can all benefit from leading a healthier lifestyle. We find evidence of Sigerist's thinking 40 years later in the Ottawa Charter for Health Promotion (WHO, 1986). This document was a response to growing expectations for a new public health movement and remains at the centre of international government thinking the world over when discussing issues of health promotion. A concept summary of the Ottawa Charter is provided below.

Concept summary: The Ottawa Charter

The Ottawa Charter for Health Promotion is the name of an international agreement signed at the First International Conference on Health Promotion, organised by the WHO and held in Ottawa, Canada, in November 1986. The charter identified three basic strategies for health promotion:

1. *Advocate.* Good health is a major resource for social, economic and personal development, and an important dimension of quality of life. Political, economic, social, cultural, environmental, behavioural and biological factors can all favour or harm health. Health promotion aims to make these conditions favourable through advocacy for health.
2. *Enable.* Health promotion focuses on achieving equity in health. Health promotion action aims to reduce differences in current health status and to ensure the availability of equal opportunities and resources to enable all people to achieve their full health potential. This includes a secure foundation in a supportive environment, access to information, life skills and opportunities to make healthy choices. People cannot achieve their fullest health potential unless they are able to control those things that determine their health. This must apply equally to women and men.
3. *Mediate.* The prerequisites and prospects for health cannot be ensured by the health sector alone. Health promotion demands co-ordinated action by all concerned, including governments, health and other social and economic sectors, non-governmental and voluntary organisations, local authorities, industry and the media.

(WHO, 1986)

Health promotion has evolved internationally over the past three decades with an emphasis on social justice, which means that each person should be treated fairly and equitably, regardless of race, age, gender or ethnicity. As a core function of public health, health promotion supports governments, communities and individuals to cope with and address health challenges.

Modern-day health promotion is largely concerned with the 'triple burden' of health constituted by communicable diseases, newly emerging and re-emerging diseases and illnesses and the unprecedented rise of people living with a long-term condition.

Communicable diseases, also known as infectious diseases or transmissible diseases, are illnesses that can be passed from person to person, and in some cases from animal to human. Some examples of communicable disease include hepatitis A, B and C, influenza, measles, Ebola and the coronavirus disease. Health promotion methods are usually aimed at preventing the spread of infection and include, among other things, the promotion of good handwashing techniques and the use of face masks.

Long-term conditions (LTCs) are defined by the Department of Health as *those conditions that cannot, at present, be cured, but can be controlled by medication and other therapies. The life of a person with an LTC is forever altered – there is no return to 'normal'* (DH, 2012, page 10). Among the most common of these conditions are asthma, diabetes, coronary heart disease, stroke, heart failure, severe mental health conditions and epilepsy. In such cases, health promotion strategies are often aimed at helping the person achieve optimal health and well-being as well as preventing the condition becoming worse.

As a nation, we are living longer but are not necessarily healthier. There are large numbers of people living with one or more long-term conditions (ONS, 2018) and the issue of frailty is high on the health promotion agenda. Nationally, life expectancy has improved year on year and there are more people living past 100 years of age than ever before. However, the health of the most disadvantaged has not improved as quickly as that of the better-off. Inequalities in health persist and, it is argued, they have widened.

The UK government has targeted its energies on five high-level enduring priorities that run through a number of national public health initiatives and national policy (e.g. DH, 2010, 2011, 2013; DHSC, 2018). These are:

1. helping people to live longer and more healthy lives by reducing preventable deaths and the burden of ill health associated with smoking, high blood pressure, obesity, poor diet, poor mental health, insufficient exercise and alcohol;

2. reducing the burden of disease and disability in life by focusing on preventing and recovering from the conditions with the greatest impact, including dementia, anxiety, depression and drug dependency;

3. protecting the country from infectious diseases and environmental hazards, including the growing problem of infections that resist treatment with antibiotics;

4. supporting families to give children and young people the best start in life, through working with health visiting and school nursing, and family–nurse partnerships;

5. improving health in the workplace by encouraging employers to support their staff, as well as those moving into and out of the workforce, to lead healthier lives.

Taken together, these targets demonstrate the complexities of meeting the changing demands of the general public, as well as their perceptions of health and what it is to be healthy.

Determinants of health

Health is heavily influenced by a number of factors that lie outside of the health-care system, especially matters relating to social justice, education, equity and public spending. These forces largely shape the circumstances in which people grow, live, work and age. Collectively, they are known as the determinants of health (Dahlgren and Whitehead, 1991). Health promotion is aimed at addressing the determinants of health, including: lifestyle factors related to individuals, such as health-related behaviours (e.g. smoking, diet, physical activity); broader factors such as income, education, employment and working conditions; and social environments such as where we live and work.

Concept summary: The determinants of health

The determinants of health include:

* the social and economic environment;
* the physical environment;
* the person's individual characteristics and behaviours.

The contexts of people's lives determine their health, and so blaming individuals for having poor health or crediting them for good health is inappropriate. Individuals are unlikely to be able to directly control many of the determinants of health. These determinants, or things that make people healthy or not, include the above factors, and many others:

* *Income and social status*: Higher income and social status are linked to better health. The greater the gap between the richest and poorest people, the greater the differences in health.
* *Education*: Low education levels are linked with poor health, more stress and lower self-confidence.
* *Physical environment*: Safe water, clean air, healthy workplaces and safe houses, communities and roads all contribute to good health.

- *Employment and working conditions:* People in employment are healthier, particularly those who have more control over their working conditions.
- *Social support networks:* Greater support from families, friends and communities is linked to better health.
- *Culture:* Customs and traditions, as well as the beliefs of the family and community, all affect health.
- *Genetics:* Inheritance plays a part in determining lifespan, healthiness and the likelihood of developing certain illnesses.
- *Personal behaviour and coping skills:* Balanced eating, keeping active, smoking, drinking and how we deal with life's stresses and challenges all affect health.
- *Health services:* Access and use of services that prevent and treat disease influence health.
- *Gender:* Men and women suffer from different types of diseases at different ages.

(WHO, 2019)

People cannot achieve their fullest health potential unless they are able to take control of those things that determine their health. Health promotion action aims at reducing differences in current health status, as well as ensuring equal opportunities and resources are available to enable all people to achieve their fullest health potential. Health promotion covers the entire lifespan of a person. This includes a secure foundation in a supportive environment, as well as access to health information, life skills and opportunities for making healthy choices in youth as in old age.

The role of the nurse

Health promotion has developed to the point that it is now considered a fundamental part of everyday nursing practice (NMC, 2018a). Nurses, regardless of their field or specialty, have an important role to play in promoting public health. Traditionally, the focus of health promotion by nurses has been on disease prevention and changing the behaviour of individuals with respect to their health.

Public Health England have developed 'All our Health Framework' (PHE, updated 2022), which is a call to action to all healthcare professionals, not just nursing, to use their knowledge, skills and relationships to work with patients and the population to prevent illness, protect health and promote well-being.

COVID-19 has further highlighted the need for nurses and other healthcare professionals to become more engaged in health promotion activities. Increasingly, health promotion is seen as crucial for our survival, not only to protect ourselves but also to protect those around us.

Gruman, Schneider and Coutts (2016) identified three levels of prevention efforts: those of primary prevention, secondary prevention and tertiary prevention. These align well with health promotion strategies following COVID-19. Primary prevention is concerned with keeping people healthy, largely through educational efforts and empowering people to take responsibility for their own health and well-being and in the case of COVID-19, the roll-out of vaccination programmes. Secondary prevention is aimed at preventing people with an existing illness or disorder from deteriorating further, and promoting recovery. For example, someone who's been diagnosed with long COVID may maintain social distancing, wear a face covering when shopping and engage in rehabilitative exercises to improve lung functioning and general fitness. Lastly, tertiary prevention is concerned with helping people with an existing, often long-term condition to achieve an optimal level of health and emotional well-being, and often involves the individual making lifestyle changes and adjustments to their thinking and outlook on life. A nurse's work environment makes it easy to take advantage of a routine interaction with a patient and their families to look at health promotion strategies in terms of primary, secondary and tertiary prevention, as well as using it as an opportunity to give information and to educate and have a health promoting conversation (see Chapter 3).

Integrated care

The need for integrated care has been defined as the bringing together of inputs, delivery, management and organisation of services related to diagnosis, treatment, care, rehabilitation and health promotion (HEE, 2019a). Integrated care takes many different forms and may involve whole populations, care for particular groups or people with the same diseases, as well as co-ordination of care for individual service users and carers. It is important that this care is co-ordinated, and that different agencies and services work together. The patient needs to know that they have the power to shape their own health and well-being, and that there is a team of people ready to support them in this. We need to see communities and people as having strengths and focus on their capabilities to manage and promote their own health and well-being, rather than focusing on problems and deficits, which often act to disempower people.

Advocating for the patient and for change

One of the very important roles of the nurse within the healthcare system is that of the patient advocate. Although this is a belief shared by nursing professionals, it is not always easy to carry out. The nurse as advocate defends patients' rights and interests, as well as assuring the safety and well-being of those who cannot advocate for themselves (Davoodvand et al., 2016). By acting as an advocate, the nurse ensures that the patient's autonomy is respected, as well as serving as a link between the patient and the healthcare system. They speak up when problems go unnoticed or when the patient or family cannot or will not address them.

Nurses, along with other professionals, voluntary and community action groups, and health personnel, have a major responsibility to mediate between differing interests in society for the pursuit of health. They can do this at the community level by running public awareness campaigns and highlighting issues by working with the mass media and taking part in national campaigns. For examples of national health and well-being campaigns, follow the link in Activity 1.1.

Activity 1.1   Critical thinking

Access the calendar of national health and well-being campaigns for 2021–2022 using the following link: www.nhsemployers.org/events/calendar-national-campaigns

This web page hosts a selection of national campaigns and awareness days for the year ahead and is regularly updated. Scroll through the site, making a note of any campaigns that are of interest to you, and then see how you can get involved. It might be that you take an event back to your nursing group or university and look to run something locally as part of a bigger campaign.

As this activity is based on your own observation, there is no outline answer at the end of the chapter.

Nurses can also help in the development of public health and health promotion policies by sitting on work committees and interest groups. Through policy work, nurses can and should influence practice standards and processes to assure quality of care. Nurses can get involved by: learning how policy is developed; learning who is participating in policy development and making contact with them; volunteering to participate in policy meetings or related activities; preparing a fact sheet; or assisting in preparing a report to inform policy decision-makers. To be influential, nurses must see themselves as professionals with the capacity and responsibility to influence current and future healthcare delivery systems, as well as recognising the important part they play in health promotion and in people's lives.

Health promotion models and theories

There are a number of significant theories and models that underpin the practice of health promotion. Theories are ideas that support a particular way of action or thought, whereas models are a means of how we might put that thinking into action. Theories and models are useful in helping us better understand the nature of the problem being addressed. They help us to describe and explain the possible needs and motivations of the people whom we are trying to support and work with. This in turn allows us to plan interventions and support people in a variety of settings relating to their behaviours and health determinants.

When identifying a theory or model to guide health promotion or disease prevention programmes, it is important to consider a range of factors, such as the specific health problem being addressed, the population(s) being served and the contexts within which the programme is being implemented.

The theoretical underpinnings for health promotion have evolved since the early 1980s. Most of these theories are behaviourally based, derived from the social sciences and extensively researched. Health promotion theories and models are often broken down into three different groups. First, there are models of change targeted at the individual. Many healthcare practitioners spend most of their work time in one-on-one activities such as counselling or patient education, and individuals are often the primary target audience for health education materials.

Second, there are theories and models that address communities and populations. Communities are often understood in geographical terms, but they can be defined by other criteria too. For instance, there are communities of shared interests (e.g. the LGBTQ+ community) or collective identity (e.g. the African British community). When planning community-level interventions, it is critical to learn about the community's unique characteristics. This is particularly true when addressing health issues in ethnically or culturally diverse communities (see Chapter 8). Comprehensive health promotion programmes often use advocacy techniques to help support individual behaviour change with organisational and regulatory change.

Third, there are new and emergent models of health promotion based around the use of communication technologies. New communication technologies have opened a wide range of avenues for influencing health behaviour (see Chapter 9), particularly the use of social media in getting a health promotion message across to a large number of people.

We will now look at some of the more popular theories and models from each of the three areas, starting with a couple of models aimed at influencing individual behaviours and thinking.

Health belief model

The health belief model (HBM) is a psychological model that attempts to explain and predict health behaviours (see Figure 1.1). This is done by focusing on the attitudes and beliefs of individuals. The HBM was first developed in the 1950s by the social psychologists Godfrey H. Hochbaum, Irwin M. Rosenstock and Stephen Kegels working in the US Public Health Service (Rosenstock, 1974). The model was developed in response to the failure of a free tuberculosis (TB) health screening programme. Since then, the HBM has been adapted to explore a variety of long- and short-term health behaviours, including sexual risk behaviours and the transmission of HIV/AIDS. It is still one of the most widely recognised and used models in health behaviour applications.

The rationale behind the HBM is that even though an individual recognises the consequences of certain health behaviours, their decisions to take action will be based on the following factors: they believe that they are susceptible to the condition (perceived susceptibility); they believe the condition has serious consequences (perceived severity);

they believe that taking action would reduce their susceptibility to the condition or its severity (perceived benefits); they believe that the costs of taking action (perceived barriers) are outweighed by the benefits; they are exposed to factors that prompt action (e.g. a television ad, a reminder from their physician to get a mammogram); and they are confident in their ability to successfully perform an action (self-efficacy). Self-efficacy refers to the extent of an individual's belief in his or her abilities (Bandura, 1997). Because self-efficacy is based on feelings of self-confidence and control, it is a good predictor of motivation and behaviour.

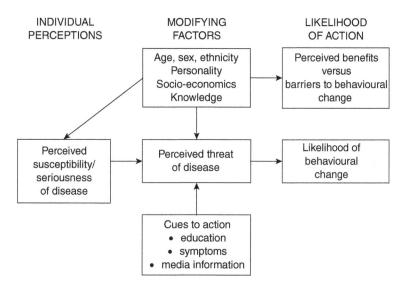

Figure 1.1   The health belief model (adapted from Glanz et al., 2002, page 52)

The HBM has been found to be most useful with preventative health behaviours such as screening and immunisation. It has been less useful in guiding interventions to address long-term, complex and socially determined behaviours such as alcohol and tobacco use (Corace et al., 2016).

Activity 1.2   Critical thinking

Think of an illness that you might have experienced. Now, using the questions below, analyse your experience in terms of the HBM:

1. Before developing the illness, had you ever thought that you were likely to develop the illness (perceived susceptibility)?
2. Had you thought that the illness was severe with possible serious complications (perceived severity)?
3. Had you considered the benefits of making lifestyle changes in response to your illness (perceived benefits) to prevent yourself from becoming ill again in the future?

(Continued)

(Continued)

4. Had you thought of any problems in making these lifestyle changes (perceived barriers)?
    Were you able to make and maintain these changes?

Because the HBM is so closely based on individual experience, it is easy to use it to think about illnesses we have had. Because of this, it helps us to understand the health beliefs of others. Repeat the exercise again, but this time think of yourself as an older person being called to get their COVID-19 vaccination.

An outline answer is provided at the end of the chapter.

Stages of change model

Developed by Prochaska and DiClemente (1983), the stages of change model evolved out of studies comparing the experiences of smokers who quit on their own with those of smokers receiving professional treatment. The model's basic premise is that behaviour change is a process to be followed; this is different to the HBM, which looks at the influences affecting a person's behaviour. Long-term changes in health behaviour involve multiple actions and adaptations over time. Some people may not be ready to attempt changes, while others may have already begun implementing changes in their lives. It is important that we understand something about where people come from in relation to making changes in their lifestyle that will promote their health. The stages of change model describe the different stages that we go through when we want to change something about ourselves or the way we live; these are pre-contemplation, contemplation, preparation, action and maintenance (see Table 1.1). Definitions of the stages vary slightly, depending on the behaviour at issue. People at different points along this continuum have different informational needs and benefit from interventions designed for their stage. It helps us to understand why some people might not be ready to attempt change and why some might be more committed to change than others.

Stage	Definition	Potential change strategies
Pre-contemplation	Has no intention of taking action within the next six months	Increase awareness of need for change; personalise information about risks and benefits
Contemplation	Intends to take action in the next six months	Motivate; encourage making specific plans
Preparation	Intends to take action within the next 30 days and has taken some behavioural steps in this direction	Assist with developing and implementing concrete action plans; help set gradual goals

| Action | Adopting new skills; has changed behaviour for less than six months | Assist with feedback, problem-solving, social support and reinforcement |
| Maintenance | Ongoing practice of new, healthier behaviour; has changed behaviour for more than six months | Assist with coping, reminders, finding alternatives and avoiding slips/relapses (as applicable) |

Table 1.1 Behaviour change stages and their characteristics

People do not always move through the stages of change in a linear manner; they often recycle and repeat certain stages (e.g. individuals may relapse and go back to an earlier stage depending on their level of motivation and self-efficacy). The stages of change model illustrates the importance of tailoring programmes to the real needs and circumstances of individuals rather than assuming an intervention will be equally applicable to all. Above all, it recognises that people are not always best placed to make changes, and individuals may not always succeed in making changes the first time.

Relapse Prevention Model

The primary emphasis of health promotion has been the initial behaviour change process. The relapse prevention model (RP) presents a strategy to enhance the likelihood of maintaining a behaviour change using methods clearly rooted in social learning theory. The widely used Marlatt and Gordon's (1985) RP model is based on social-cognitive and behavioural strategies to prevent or limit relapse episodes. Central to the model is the detailed classification of factors or situations that can precipitate or contribute to relapse episodes. These generally fall within two categories: 1) immediate determinants (e.g. high-risk situations, a person's coping skills, outcome expectations, etc.) and 2) covert antecedents (e.g. lifestyle imbalances, urges and cravings). The relapse prevention model employs strategies to help build an awareness that helps the person understand the types of situations that could trigger a relapse and then helps people learn better ways to cope with these triggers and reduce the risk of relapse.

Pender's Health Promotion Model

The Health Promotion Model was designed by Nola Pender, a former professor of nursing at the University of Michigan. Written with the nurse in mind, it was to be a *complementary counterpart to models of health protection* (1982; revised 1996). Pender's Health Promotion Model aims to explain the factors underlying motivation to engage in health promoting behaviours and focuses on people's interactions with their physical and interpersonal environments during attempts to improve health. The model focuses on three areas:

- individual characteristics and experiences;
- behaviour-specific cognitions and affect;
- behaviour outcomes.

The model emphasises the active role that a person has in initiating and maintaining health promoting behaviour, and in shaping their own environment to support health promoting behaviours. It makes four assumptions; these are:

1. Individuals seek to actively control their own behaviour.

2. Individuals interact with their environment, progressively transforming the environment as well as being transformed by it over time.

3. Health professionals, such as nurses, constitute a part of the interpersonal environment, which exerts influence on people throughout their lifespan.

4. The way in which we relate to our environment and those in it is essential to changing behaviour.

The model concentrates on three categories: individual categories and experiences, behaviour-specific cognitions and affect, and the behavioural outcomes. The first category looks at how each individual has their own set of characteristics and experiences, which in turn shape their actions and behaviours.

The second category involves the behaviour-specific cognitions and affect (the way the person thinks and feels) which have a direct impact on the individual's motivation for change.

The third category is the behavioural outcome. By making a start the person commits to making a change. During this phase the person is supported in tackling barriers to change. The desired behaviour and whether it is reached is influenced by the immediate competing demand and preferences of the person, which can derail intended actions for promoting health. Health behavioural change is the result of reciprocal relationships among the environment, personal factors and attributes of the behaviour itself. The goal of the Pender Health Promotion Model is to simulate a behavioural change that results in a positive outcome.

Diffusion of innovation theory

While the models in the first group apply to individual behaviour, the models in the second group are directed at understanding and improving the health of populations rather than focusing on the health of individuals.

The diffusion of innovation model was first introduced in 1962 by Everett Rogers. The model is not specific to health innovations but pertains to all innovations. Rogers (1983) defines diffusion as *the process by which an innovation is communicated through certain channels over time among the members of a social system* (page 5). By identifying the variables that will determine how an innovation is taken up by different members of a community, these types of models assist health promoters in planning how to introduce a new idea or practice into the community. According to Rogers (1983), a number of factors determine how quickly, and to what extent, an innovation will be adopted and diffused:

- The relative advantage of an innovation shows its superiority over whatever it replaces.
- Compatibility is an appropriate fit with the intended audience.
- Complexity has to do with how easy it is to implement the innovation.
- Trialability pertains to whether it can be tried on an experimental basis.
- Observability reflects whether the innovation will produce tangible results.

Effective diffusion requires practitioners to use both informal and formal communication channels and a spectrum of strategies for different settings. Disseminating an innovation in a variety of ways increases the likelihood that it will be adopted. To be effective, the behaviour must be promoted on multiple levels, in multiple settings, using multiple strategies. Once a critical number of individuals in a population have adopted the behaviour, the adoption process becomes self-sustaining.

Communities work differently from hierarchies and government administrations. With time, they develop their own implicit and explicit systems. These systems reflect the different interests, conflicts and priorities that change with time and with generations. Accordingly, the skills, knowledge, values and practice of the community also change with time. The pace at which the community develops differs from that at which health services evolve. Thus, matching community development with health service development is complex, and more so with each new generation.

Theories of organisational change

Theories of organisational change assist health promoters in understanding how change occurs within organisations and in planning for this. The stage theory of organisational change (Lewin, 1951; Robertson et al., 1993) is probably the best known of the organisational development change theories and has stood the test of time. It helps to explain how organisations plan and implement new ways of working and looks at, among other things, how quality of life at work might be promoted (e.g. achieving a healthy work–life balance). The stage theory of organisational change can be said to consist of four stages:

1. *Awareness*: Problems are recognised and analysed, and solutions suggested and evaluated.
2. *Adoption*: Policies are formulated, and resources for beginning change(s) are allocated.
3. *Implementation*: The innovation is implemented, reactions take place, and changes in roles occur.
4. *Institutionalisation*: The policy or programme becomes an integral part of the organisation, and new goals and values are a part of its structure (e.g. all members of staff get off on time).

The success of such programmes, it is hoped, will bring about systemic and lasting change within and have positive health benefits.

Communication theory

The third category looks at approaches and thinking that guide the use of communication strategies in public health and health promotion. Focused on improving the health of communities rather than examining the underlying processes of communication, public health communication is the scientific development, strategic dissemination and evaluation of relevant, accurate, accessible and understandable health information, communicated to and from intended audiences to advance the public's health (WHO, 2017).

Public health policy and initiatives are increasingly being promoted through the use of social and mass media. Using a variety of communication channels can allow health messages to shape mass media or interpersonal, small group or community-level campaigns. Health communication strategies aim to change people's knowledge, attitudes and/or behaviours by increasing risk perception, reinforcing positive behaviours, influencing social norms (e.g. having open discussions about safe sex), increasing the availability of support and needed services, and empowering individuals to change or improve their health conditions through information and education. Activity 1.3 encourages you to explore a successful media campaign aimed at helping people to stop smoking.

Activity 1.3   Research

Here is an example of an online public health campaign, Stoptober, aimed at stopping smoking. Take time to explore the site and visit the links: **www.blf.org.uk/take-action/campaign-with-us/stoptober**

- Consider how the website is presented.
- How accessible is the site to navigate?
- How have personal stories of giving up smoking been used in support of the overall campaign?

As this activity is based on your own observation, there is no outline answer at the end of the chapter.

Media campaigns of this kind draw on social marketing techniques and understanding. Social marketing is the application of commercial marketing techniques, such as market analysis, to the health and welfare context (Bhat, Darzi & Hakim, 2019). Combining ideas from commercial marketing and the social sciences, social marketing is a proven tool for influencing behaviour.

Four questions figure largely when using a social marketing approach to health promotion:

1. Do I really understand my target audience and see things from their perspective?

2. Am I clear about what I would like my target audience to do?

3. For my target audience, do the benefits of doing what I would like them to do outweigh the costs or barriers to doing it?

4. Am I using a combination of activities in order to encourage people to achieve the desired action?

Concept summary: Communication technologies

New communication technologies have opened an extraordinary range of avenues for influencing health behaviour. The advent of social media and advancement in communication technologies have really challenged the way we think about how we communicate and disseminate public health messages, information and education. The benefits that new technologies bring include:

*   increased reach (the ability to communicate to broad, geographically dispersed audiences);
*   asynchronous communication (interaction not bounded by having to communicate at the same time);
*   the ability to integrate multiple communication modes and formats (e.g. audio, video, text, graphics);
*   the ability to track, preserve and analyse communication (e.g. computer records of interaction, analysis of interaction trends);
*   user control of the communication system (the ability to customise programmes to user specifications);
*   interactivity (e.g. increased capacity for feedback).

(Welch et al., 2016)

The rise of public and social media has undoubtedly had an impact on their popularity as an intervention, with health and lifestyle information and advice never more than a few clicks away. However, the use of communication technologies can also have disadvantages, some of which are listed below:

*   inequity in access;
*   navigational challenges;
*   poor-quality health information resulting in the person adopting harmful behaviours;
*   patient isolation and feeling of abandonment;
*   risk related to breach of protected health information.

Chapter summary

Over the last four decades, the field of health promotion has emerged and provided a new way of thinking about the root causes of health and well-being. Health promotion is complex and works on a number of levels, and this is reflected in the health promotion theories and models discussed. Health promotion is directed towards action on the determinants of health, and combines diverse, but complementary, methods and approaches.

Practising health promotion requires the nurse to think about the interactions they have with those whom they look after and care for, as well as viewing their patients in a holistic way. Health promotion is not just about treating illness and disease; it is also about helping people to achieve optimum health and maintain good health for as long as they can. It is about promoting positive health for all.

Activities: Brief outline answers

Activity 1.2 Critical thinking (page 17)

1. *Perceived susceptibility:* The flu vaccination campaign is aimed at anyone aged 65 or over, and therefore the older person might perceive themselves at risk of catching flu.

2. *Perceived severity:* Flu is more severe in older people and adults with an underlying health condition, such as long-term heart or respiratory disease. The older person with one of these conditions might worry about how catching flu might affect their existing health problems.

3. *Perceived benefits:* The flu vaccine helps to prevent people from getting the flu; if they do get it, their symptoms are reduced.

4. *Perceived barriers:* The older person might rely on public transport. Making an appointment and getting to the GP to have their flu vaccination might prove difficult.

Further reading

Willis, J (2022) *Foundations for Health Promotion*, 5th edition. London: Elsevier.

This book, written by one of the leading writers on health promotion, discusses health promotion theories in greater depth than we can do here.

Useful website

https://campaignresources.phe.gov.uk/resources/campaigns

The Public Health England Resource Centre lists the many Health Promotion campaigns currently being run in the UK and provides a useful insight into the breadth, depth and diversity of such activities.

Chapter 2   Core skills for health promotion

Chapter aims

After reading this chapter, you will be able to:

- identify the core skills required of the nurse to carry out a health promotion intervention;
- understand the principles of effective communication techniques when delivering health promotion activities in the healthcare setting;
- discuss the value and nature of the nurse–patient relationship when carrying out a health promotion conversation;
- begin working with patients on making choices about their health and well-being.

Introduction

This chapter will look at the fundamental skills required of the nurse to successfully deliver health promotion activities when working with individuals and their families. It starts by outlining the skills required of the nurse before exploring each in greater detail. It then looks at how these skills might be employed in clinical practice. In doing this, the chapter explores the challenges and barriers faced by nurses providing public health interventions and the many ways in which the nurse can promote and help protect good health and well-being through the nurse–patient relationship. The chapter ends with a summary of the key points and ideas for taking these skills forward into practice.

Case study: Jack

Jack is a 48-year-old man who, except for hypertension, considers himself healthy. He saw his family doctor three months ago for a regular blood pressure check-up, as he does every six months. Jack is married, has four adolescent children, and has worked as a car sales-man for the last 14 years. He leads a rather sedentary lifestyle. Jack's wife, Sarah, is worried about the *amount of weight Jack has put on during COVID-19, when Jack was working from home a lot of the time.* At 6 ft, 3 in, Jack is a tall man. He has a BMI of 32.0 and is obese. He has a waist circumference of 52 in. By his own admission, he does not eat the best of diets and enjoys 'fatty foods', such as crisps and sausage rolls. Sarah has tried to introduce 'more vegetables into their diet' and encourage them both to lead a 'healthier lifestyle', but to no effect. Jack is to go into hospital to have an **arthroscopy** of the knee. During preparation for theatre, concern has been expressed as to Jack's weight and hypertension given that he is to receive a general anaesthetic. Jack is keen that the operation is not postponed, having been cancelled several times already owing to COVID-19 restrictions.

The nurse has been asked to have a health conversation with Jack about his weight. The nurse recognises that she has a duty to promote health where she can, although she is not altogether comfortable talking to people about their weight.

The following case study: Alexis also contains the opportunity to have a health promotion conversation. While there is concern about the young person's weight, the context is quite different and there is the suggestion that Alexis's mental health might have been negatively impacted by her experiences of COVID-19. There is also the opportunity to have a health-promoting conversation with Alexis's stepfather, who is attempting to give up smoking.

Case study: Alexis

Alexis is a 14-year-old female who was diagnosed with asthma four years ago by her asthma nurse specialist at her GP surgery. Alexis lives at home with her mother, stepfather and younger brother. Alexis suffers with eczema and seasonal allergic rhinitis (SAR) during the summer months, resulting in hay fever symptoms. Furthermore, at the time of her diagnosis, the main triggers for her asthma included undertaking exercise, exposure to cats and frequent respiratory tract infections.

Alexis's mother is worried that Alexis uses a lot of hand sanitiser to avoid COVID-19 and catching 'other infections' and has taken to isolating herself and spending many hours in her bedroom alone. Alexis is also 'putting on weight' as she is not exercising or socialising. Alexis's stepfather is a smoker but her mother states he smokes outside and is trying at the moment to quit.

During the pandemic, health promotion focused on helping people maintain a healthy lifestyle, particularly during lockdown. At the start of the pandemic, empowerment and self-care were promoted, while healthcare provision rapidly shifted to COVID-19 prevention and care. As we learn to live with COVID-19, health promotion has taken centre stage by enabling people to increase control over their health. Nurses need to understand their role in health promotion and the skills that go with this.

The nature of health promotion skills

Nurses are increasingly aware that although there is a lot they can do to help their patients, there is much more that patients can do to help themselves. The goal of any nursing care, not just health promotion, should be to maximise the individual's capabilities to look after their own health, promote a level of wellness and enhance their independence. In order to do this, the nurse adopts what is known as a person-centred approach. In using a person-centred approach, we have the following goals:

- to encourage patients to express concerns, fears and expectations;
- to help them to be more active in the consultation;
- to allow them to articulate what information they require;
- to give them greater control of decision making, and therefore responsibility, particularly when talking about changes in their behaviour;
- to reach decisions jointly and ensure that goals are feasible.

(Mason and Butler, 2010)

In using a person-centred approach, the nurse encourages the person to express any concerns, fears and expectations that they may have regarding their health and well-being. This assists the person in articulating what information they require and what support they may need going forward. In doing so, the nurse focuses on what is important to the person and respects their wishes when planning and managing their care. Wherever possible, any decision regarding the person's care should be reached jointly. The nurse helps the person to explore their thoughts, feelings and behaviour towards a particular topic or issue, and by doing so reaches a clear understanding of what the person is going through.

Health promotion skills

Health promotion is concerned with fostering the motivation, skills and confidence necessary for the person to take action to improve their health and well-being. Health promotion may be seen as the process whereby one person enables another to constructively resolve personal problem(s) that may be long-standing or acute. This process requires the nurse to help others find their own strengths to cope more effectively with their lives. The nurse can help the person achieve this by supporting them in their decision making, encouraging them to look at alternative ways of acting and getting them to evaluate the consequences of these actions. Behaviours that have met with success should be celebrated and built upon.

The skills required to carry out a health promotion intervention can be broken down into three broad areas: (1) the ability to engage and communicate with people; (2) the ability to show empathy and encourage others; and (3) skills in listening and questioning. These in turn require the nurse to be able to think creatively, use problem-solving skills and be flexible in their approach when dealing with people. These will now be explored in greater depth.

The ability to engage and communicate with people

The ability to engage and communicate with people is fundamental to all nursing care, not only health promotion. The wanting and willingness to engage with people is the starting point of all healthcare interventions. It is through positive engagement that we foster an understanding of the person and what they are going through. Engagement is the demonstration of willingness to become involved and pursue an understanding of the patient's situation as they see it (WHO, 2016). Engagement lays the groundwork for what follows and builds trust between people. Active engagement with another means putting them first in all that we do. Engagement is indicated by the way we conduct ourselves and the way in which we talk and respond to the patient. For example, if you work on the principle that patients are to have as much **autonomy** as possible, it is not appropriate to force our views upon them, however much you may have their interests at heart, or act to exclude them because they do not agree with what you have to say. It is important to understand what drives our conversations. Activity 2.1 asks you to reflect on this.

Activity 2.1 Reflection

Reflect back on a conversation you had with someone about their health, and ask yourself the following questions:

1. What was my motivation in starting the conversation?
2. What was my intention in pursuing the conversation?
3. Was I just following a role, completing a task, or was I genuinely interested in what the other person had to say?

As this activity is based on your own experience, there is no outline answer at the end of the chapter.

The process of engagement is enhanced by the use of an empathic approach (Jeffery, 2016). Empathy means being in touch with another person and having an understanding of what they are going through at that moment. Responding in an empathic way means involvement; it is not a passive activity. Rather than denying the other person's experience, you encourage them to share what is troubling them, accepting them and not evaluating them as a person. The idea behind a health- promoting conversation is to:

- meaningfully engage with the person;
- build trust;
- focus on raising the other's awareness and self-knowledge by asking questions;
- focus on solutions and not problems;
- be a strong ally, who encourages the other when needed;
- help the other unlock their potential by inspiring new ideas and encouraging creativity.

Communication skills

Effective communication is one of the ways in which we demonstrate empathy and understanding of the person. To have someone who will help the person look at issues and support them without taking over can be very powerful indeed. Sometimes all the nurse has to do is co-ordinate and make available the resources required to bring about the change, or simply let another person know where to find these resources themselves. Occasionally, the nurse will suggest solutions. However, all this requires communication and an understanding of the person.

Health promoting communication engages individuals in conversations that increase clarity, improve understanding of the situation and provide impetus for change. In order to do this, the nurse must process good listening skills, as well as the ability to move a conversation on through raising the other's awareness and self-knowledge by asking questions.

Listening skills

The most common way we communicate understanding is by listening to what the other person is telling us. Listening refers to the interpretative process that takes place with what we hear. It involves attention, interpretation and understanding. When we listen, we do not just sit passively while the other person talks; we actively let them know that they are being attended to, heard and understood. Effective listening is an empathic and caring act that will let the other person know that you understand and accept them.

Active listening means, as the name suggests, actively listening to what the other person has to say and how they say it. Truly listening to a person is a skill that requires thought, attention, time and effort. By actively listening, individuals feel understood and valued, and are more likely to disclose information and be more open in what they say. This can lead to increased insight and open up the opportunity for problem solving and creative thinking. By being willing to enter into a dialogue, even with people with whom you disagree or are lacking in motivation, you will be able to have more honest and productive conversations.

Active listening requires an open and honest curiosity about the other person, as well as a willingness and ability to keep the spotlight on them. This can mean thinking beyond the words, listening to what lies behind surface meaning and carefully observing body language. The more interested and focused you are, the more animated the person is likely to be, as well as interested in you and what you have to say. Create an environment that will allow both of you to focus with minimum interruptions and distractions. Be patient and do not interrupt unnecessarily. Pauses in the conversation can be very useful, so give the person time to pause and reflect. Allowing the person the gift of time to explain their position and pursue their thoughts allows the nurse to apprehend information in context, and therefore understand the person and their behaviour better.

Active listening is supported and enhanced by the use of attending behaviours (see Table 2.1). Attending behaviours are all forms of non-verbal communication, such as eye contact, body posture and behaviours (e.g. sitting on the same level as the patient, leaning towards the patient, encouraging gestures, nodding in agreement), which demonstrate that you are interested in what the patient has to say. A nurse can encourage a patient to continue to talk and explore issues in greater depth through active listening and attending behaviours.

An effective verbal communicator:	An effective non-verbal communicator:
• Clarifies (the problem) • Listens (actively) • Encourages (empathically) • Acknowledges (the person and what they are going through) • Rephrases/Reflects (understanding)	• Relaxes • Opens up • Leans towards the other person • Establishes eye contact • Shows appropriate facial expressions

Table 2.1   Characteristics of an effective communicator (CLEAR ROLES)

There are a number of beneifits to actively listening and engaging with a person. Individuals feel understood and valued and are more likely to disclose information and be more open to offers of help. Likewise, individuals feel that they are being offered an opportunity to state their thoughts and feelings more clearly. This can lead to increased insight and open up the opportunity for problem solving and creative thinking.

Paraphrasing, reflecting and summarising

Paraphrasing, reflecting and summarising are three more ways of communicating to the person that they have been listened to, and are skills used in counselling.

Paraphrasing is not a matter of simply repeating what the person has had to say but capturing the essence of what the person is saying, through rephrasing. When the nurse has captured what the person is saying, often the person will say, 'That's right' or offer some other feedback of confirmation. Reflection is a form of paraphrasing that is generally limited to feelings. The purpose of reflection in this situation is to process and make meaning of what the person is saying. This not only means listening to what the person has to say, but also what feelings and emotions the person is experiencing when sharing their story with you. Reflecting is to show an understanding and acceptance of what the person is going through. It also allows the person to make sure that you fully understood them; if not, they can correct you. Summarising allows you to check in with the person that you actually do understand what has been said, and it gives the person an opportunity to clarify any points – sometimes the clarification is for the other person's benefit as much as your own.

Asking questions and providing prompts

Questions may be used to open conversations and initiate social interaction. They may also be used to elicit personal and medical information, to ascertain attitudes, opinions and feelings, to show interest in a topic or another person, to identify needs, to assess a person's knowledge and understanding, to help conversations go smoothly, to encourage exploration of experiences and to direct action. In health promotion conversations, asking questions can help to open up new areas for discussion. How you ask questions, as well as the questions you choose, are really important. You should ask questions in an inquisitive manner, not in a challenging way. Do not show approval or disapproval in your questions but display a friendly neutrality. Show curiosity and a desire to learn about the person's position. As a nurse, you can (and probably will) influence a patient, but you should take the view that the best ideas will actually come from the patient. One of the most powerful tools a nurse has is their ability to ask questions that encourage the patient to take a different perspective and resolve issues for themselves. A good question is simple, has purpose, and is influencing but not controlling.

The way in which a question is asked in part determines how well it serves the function that was intended. Much of the research into the verbal behaviour of nurses indicates that nurses tend to use inappropriate styles of questioning that result in failures of communication from both their own and the patient's point of view (Fitzpatrick, 2018). Patients are not given the opportunity to explore their feelings, while nurses fail to detect underlying needs and frequently miss the opportunity to gather vital information.

There are two main types of questions: open and closed. To find out about a patient's situation and the issues they face, as well as helping them to find answers, use more open questions than closed. Closed questions are ones that limit the possibilities of reply. They are used in the collection of facts and to discover preferences between given alternatives; frequently, they invite yes/no answers, and thus do not encourage much talk.

Open questions are those that cannot be answered in a few words; they encourage the patient to speak and offer an opportunity for the nurse to gather information about the patient and their concerns. They encourage talk as yes/no answers are difficult to give. Because the focus is on the person to provide detail, the conversation and its direction are much more in their hands. As the content of the reply is unpredictable, the nurse needs considerable skill in picking up cues in order to pursue the conversation meaningfully, as well as to avoid becoming sidetracked.

Open questions are particularly valuable in eliciting attitudes, values, opinions and feelings, and as such may be threatening to either party. This can mean rethinking old attitudes, challenging current practices and finding ways of being creative and innovative. Typically, open questions begin with 'what', 'when', 'who', 'why' and 'how'. For example:

1. What has brought you here today?
2. Why do you think that?
3. How did you come to consider this?
4. Could you develop your exercise routine?
5. When do you see yourself completing the form?

'What' questions more often lead to the emergence of facts. 'Why' questions can provoke feelings of defensiveness in the person and may encourage them to feel as though they need to justify themselves in some way, and the nurse should limit their use of such questions. 'How' questions tend to invite the person to talk about their feelings. 'When' questions bring about information regarding the problem, and this can include events and information preceding or following the event. 'Where' questions usually give the nurse information regarding the reasons for the event or information leading up to an event.

Qualities of a powerful question

There is a skill and art to asking the right question at the right time. The right questions help people to articulate just what it is they want, as well as find answers and solutions to their problems. A powerful question gets the person thinking. By asking a powerful question, the nurse invites the person to clarify their thinking and behaviour and open up action and discovery at a whole new level. Examples of powerful questions include: What are your options? How do you explain this to yourself? What do you plan to do about this? What are the possible solutions? Where do you want to go from here? What are your expectations of me, the nurse? A powerful question is usually a single question – not multiple questions wrapped up in a single sentence. A powerful question is never a closed one but an open-ended one that invites reflection. Powerful questions are real questions, not advice in disguise and come from a sincere curiosity and respect. They are not leading to a particular outcome but prompt thinking about the issue being discussed. As you engage in health promotion conversations look to make a note of what questions you asked that brought about success and a change in thinking; it's likely that these were powerful questions.

Prompts

Prompts can be given in the form of questions when the person has become stuck. These are sometimes expressed as statements. They are useful when the person has dried up or if you think there is more the person could tell you about something. Examples of prompts are as follows:

- Tell me a bit more about that.
- Describe that for me.
- Tell me how you felt when you started your presentation.
- Can you give me a specific example?
- What happened next?
- How did that make you feel?
- How else might you have dealt with that?

Prompts are useful for getting the person to expand the topic out after a short response, or for encouraging them to think more about a situation or experience. They help you get at what is not being said or to find out more detail, and in turn give you a greater understanding of what the person is going through.

Holding a health promoting conversation is essentially a practical exercise and while it might look straightforward it is incredibly complex. You will find that your skill at holding such a conversation will get better with practice. No two situations are the same and what works for one individual may not necessarily work for another. Being flexible in how we approach and engage with a person is another important skill.

Shared decision making

There are times when the most helpful thing a nurse can do for someone else who has a problem is to provide the sort of conditions which will encourage that person to explore the problem and arrive at viable solutions for themselves. In these situations, persuasion is no good, reassurance is difficult, and advice-giving is inappropriate (see Chapter 1). Open questions are used frequently in conjunction with reflective listening skills in order to establish empathy and create an accepting environment in which the person can explore an issue troubling to them. By exploring the patient's ideas, concerns and expectations (ICE), you get a true understanding of where the patient is coming from (Matthys et al., 2009):

- Patient's *ideas*: 'Had you any thoughts about what might be going on?'
- Patient's *concerns*: 'And what particular worries or concerns did you have?'
- Patient's *expectations*: 'And what are you hoping to change?'

Keep in mind that during your conversations, the focus should be entirely on the patient, and that what you might think, or what your solutions for them might be, should remain unsaid. This is not something that will come naturally to most people. It is easy to fall into the trap of making assumptions, thinking you know more about the patient's health and well-being than you do, and asking questions that lead, direct or control them. The risk is that at best, the patient will give you the answers they believe you want to hear rather than what they really think or feel, and at worst you may alienate them and lose rapport. Good verbal communication means saying just enough – do not talk too much or too little. It is also worth remembering that there will be times when you do not keep on asking questions but allow periods of silence. Give the patient the time they need to think about and then answer a question. You might even say, 'Take your time' or, 'Really think about this'. Don't just jump in to break the silence if it seems to be taking a while, but be observant, read the signs and realise when the patient is not going to say more.

Involving people in their own health and care requires services to shift the focus of support from 'What is the matter with you?' to 'What matters to you?' Unlike some other healthcare interventions that emphasise the nurse as an authority figure, health promotion strategies recognise that the true power for change rests within the patient. Self-efficacy, or a belief in your own abilities to deal with various situations, can play a role in not only how you feel about yourself, but whether or not you successfully achieve your goals in life. Self-efficacy also determines what goals we choose to pursue, how we go about accomplishing those goals, and how we reflect upon our own performance. A person who feels confident that they will lose weight by attending a slimmers' club is more likely to commit to losing weight than one who believes they will never lose weight despite the support and help of others. Ultimately, it is up to the person to follow through with making changes happen. This is empowering to the individual, but also gives them responsibility for their actions. Activity 2.2 asks you to consider how you might facilitate this.

Activity 2.2 Reflection

Think of the conversations you currently have with patients and their families, and ask yourself:

1. Is the patient reliant upon me to tell them what to do?
2. Are the goals mine or theirs?
3. Am I listening more or talking more?

The chances are that if the patient is reliant on you to tell them what to do, if their care goals are yours and not theirs, and if you are doing more of the talking, then you are working in a way that disempowers, rather than empowers, the patient. If this is the case, then you might look to shift the focus of your conversations.

As this activity is based on your own observation, there is no outline answer at the end of the chapter.

Giving praise

Lastly, people usually prefer to be liked and appreciated by others. It is enhancing for them to be told what they are doing well and what you appreciate about them. If you want someone to continue to behave in a particular way, then the best way of encouraging or reinforcing that behaviour is to give acknowledgement and praise when it occurs. Remember, the purpose of praise is to help people understand what to do more of, what success looks like and what is valued. However, be careful not to overdo it as this can seem false and possibly patronising.

Chapter summary

This chapter has looked at the key components and skills for holding a health promotion conversation. This is centred on the notion of empowerment and respect for patient autonomy. Not only does this acknowledge the individual as an expert in their own care, but it also gives people greater choice and control over the care and support they receive. Holding a health promotion conversation is essentially a practical exercise, and you will find that your skill at holding such conversations will get better with practice. No two situations are identical, and what works within one relationship will not necessarily work for another. In holding a health promotion conversation, we use a combination of questioning, listening, observation and feedback to create a conversation that is rich in insight and learning. In this way, health and well-being needs are better met and people are supported to manage their health, as well as the impact it has on their lives, more effectively.

Further reading

Health Education England (HEE) (2017) *Person-Centred Approaches: Empowering People in Their Lives and Communities to Enable an Upgrade in Prevention, Well-Being, Health, Care and Support.* London: HEE.

This framework was introduced to support person-centred approaches for those working in health and social care settings. The framework helps workers to communicate meaningfully, both verbally and non-verbally, tailoring the care and advice they give to suit people's needs. It supports individuals to better manage their own health and well-being through bespoke care, planning and support. Where appropriate, the framework encourages shared decision making, outlining all reasonable options, and ensuring that all information is personalised, accessible and useful.

Useful websites

www.ausmed.co.uk/guides/communication-skills

This web page is housed on the Ausmed website, which offers free online training in the fundamental skills of nursing.

www.skillsforhealth.org.uk/wp-content/uploads/2021/01/Person-Centred-Approaches-Framework.pdf

This link takes you to the Skills for Health Person Centred Approaches Framework, which provides some useful strategies when thinking about conversations to engage, enable and support people.

www.guidelinesinpractice.co.uk/your-practice/top-tips-using-motivational-interviewing-strategies/456768.article

This site provides a number of top tips for using motivational interviewing strategies as part of clinical practice.

Chapter 3 Making every contact count (MECC)

Chapter aims

After reading this chapter, you will be able to:

- identify the key elements that make up a Making Every Contact Count (MECC) conversation;
- demonstrate an awareness and understanding of the challenges that people face when making decisions about their health and well-being;
- explain and describe the use of behaviour change approaches to empower people to manage their own health and well-being;
- demonstrate an awareness of your own communication skills to support others in making positive health choices.

Introduction

This chapter starts with a case study to help illustrate the difficulties that people have when talking about their health, including nurses. Treating people without identifying and changing what makes them unwell can be self-defeating. This thinking has sparked the development of new approaches to improving the health of individuals and communities. This chapter looks at one such initiative, that of making every contact count (MECC). It starts by giving an overview of MECC before looking at its component parts. It looks at the evidence base for MECC and why it has proved so successful. It then explains how to conduct an MECC conversation building on the skills discussed in the previous chapter, before ending with a summary of the key points.

Case study: Michael and Jenny

Michael is a 59-year-old man who has smoked since the age of 14. Like many smokers, he is not happy with his habit and would like to stop. He has booked in to see the GP practice nurse in order to get some help and advice. He has had a morning cough for about ten years and has lately noticed that although he can walk for long distances on the flat, he struggles to walk up slight inclines at anything but a slow pace. He has been trying to pass this off as an ageing process, but he is now unable to keep up with his wife and other friends of a similar age. He fears that his breathing problems may be smoking-related, having recently seen a series of TV adverts.

He is worried that his practice nurse might consider his illness to be 'self-inflicted', but he defends this by explaining to himself that he started smoking at a young age when it was common and accepted as the norm among his friends and family. He remembers that there were adverts actively encouraging you to smoke at the time he was growing up.

Jenny is a second-year adult student nurse on placement with the practice nurse. Jenny, who is to sit in on the consultation, is not looking forward to the 'inevitable' conversation on stopping smoking, as she is a smoker herself. She knows it is wrong to smoke and has tried giving up, but without success. While she is uncomfortable with such conversations, she is keen to hear what the practice nurse has to suggest and hopes to get some new ideas about stopping smoking. She would never consider asking someone 'in the profession' for help, as she 'thinks she should know better'.

Making every contact count (MECC)

Making every contact count (MECC) is a term used to describe the mechanism of brief advice and behaviour change interventions (Collins, 2015). At its heart, it seeks to make the most of the many contacts that health and social care staff have with those whom they look after and care for, as well as using those contacts as opportunities to hold positive health conversations. MECC was designed, introduced and promoted as a means of encouraging and helping people to make healthier choices to achieve positive long-term behaviour change. It draws on behavioural science research which suggests that brief interventions can be effective in producing small but important changes in behaviour, particularly if the intervention is motivational in content and offers a degree of hope for the person going forward.

Making changes such as stopping smoking, improving diet, increasing physical activity, losing weight and reducing alcohol consumption can all help people to reduce their risk of poor health as well as have a positive effect on a person's sense of mental well-being. MECC is based on the simple premise that what people do in their everyday lives – what they eat, how much they exercise and how far they follow advice on maintaining a healthy lifestyle – largely determines their health and their need for healthcare (WHO, 2006). The intention behind MECC is to help people make positive choices about their health and well-being, as well as aiming to help people develop a healthy lifestyle. For example, it can include advice on low- or no-cost activity, such as persuading parents to walk their children to school, or, as part of physical activity advice, encouraging increased use of existing community resources such as leisure centres and swimming pools. It does this by building capacity and confidence in people to make change, by supporting them in making lifestyle decisions about their own health, setting health goals and effecting change. It aims to help people to take more responsibility for their health and take early action to prevent or delay illness. This may involve addressing lifestyle areas such as poor sexual health or taking practical steps such as being immunised against contracting hepatitis B. It may also involve ensuring that individuals can access services to support the wider determinants of health (see Chapter 1), such as housing or financial support, which may be barriers to making healthy lifestyle choices. Even if the person has an existing medical condition, such as type 2 diabetes or coronary heart disease, then adopting a healthier lifestyle can make a big difference to how well the person recovers and how they manage their health into the future.

Although innovations have been developed by a number of localities, MECC's origins are in work done by NHS Yorkshire and the Humber (2010), which aimed to ensure that NHS staff used every opportunity to help patients and visitors make informed choices about their health-related behaviours, lifestyles and health services. This model was in turn based on the National Institute for Health and Care Excellence (NICE) public health guidance on promoting health-related behaviour change (NICE, 2007). MECC was championed at the NHS Future Forum (2012), who made the recommendation that every healthcare organisation should deliver MECC and *build the prevention of poor health and promotion of healthy living into their day-to-day business*. This message was reinforced in the MECC consensus statement issued by Public Health England (PHE, 2016) and included in the *NHS Standard Contract 2017/19* (NHS England, 2016). The latter made it a legal requirement that providers of health develop and maintain an organisational plan to ensure that staff use every contact they have with service users and the public as an opportunity to maintain or improve health and well-being.

> ## Activity 3.1   Critical thinking
>
> Thinking about Michael's situation in the case study above, consider why people may be reluctant to talk about their health and well-being. Michael has smoked for a long time. Can you think of some reasons why Michael may not want to talk about his concerns regarding his health?
>
> *An outline answer is provided at the end of the chapter.*

Michael may have many reasons for giving up smoking, only some of which he shares at the meeting. The decision to stop smoking, like the decision to engage in any health-related behaviour, is a complex process that is subject to a number of influences (e.g. a person's belief in their ability to give up a particular activity or lifestyle). Michael's inability to keep up when walking with family and friends, advertisements to quit smoking on television and concern for his health led to him booking an appointment with the practice nurse. Activity 3.1 asked you to reflect on Michael's reasons for stopping smoking and seeking help. Activity 3.2 asks you to explore the same situation but this time from Jenny's perspective.

> ## Activity 3.2   Reflection
>
> Reflecting on the case study at the beginning of the chapter, but this time from Jenny's perspective, discuss the following points with your peers and mentor:
>
> *   Do nurses have the right to judge people who lead unhealthy lifestyles?
> *   Should nurses who do not pursue a healthy lifestyle be in a position to give advice to patients about how to manage their health?
> *   Should nurses act as role models to the public by adopting and maintaining healthy lifestyles (e.g. not smoking, drinking in moderation, taking regular exercise)?
>
> *As this activity is based on your own reflections, there is no outline answer at the end of the chapter.*

It is not for Jenny or the nurse to judge Michael's reasons for wanting to stop smoking, but to support him in doing so. Smoking cessation is most successful if the person decides that they should stop and then takes the next step of stopping or seeking help. We should seek to understand the reasons for the person wanting to stop or change a behaviour.

MECC should be a conversation that honours autonomy and is grounded in the point of view and experiences of the person. It is important to remember that MECC is not about telling people what to do, but empowering people to make informed choices as to how they lead their lives. It involves enhancing, identifying and acting on the opportunities to engage people in conversations about their health in a respectful way to help them take action for their own health and well-being.

Having an MECC conversation

Having an MECC lifestyle conversation can be broken down into six parts:

1. spotting opportunities to talk to people about their well-being;
2. being able and confident to start a conversation about a well-being matter;
3. being able and confident to deal with any issues that arise;
4. quickly assessing the motivation a person has to take action to improve their well-being (e.g. taking a small step that will help them);
5. providing information to take action themselves;
6. signposting to relevant services when required.

The COVID-19 pandemic had a profound effect on the way people communicated and sought help. Lockdown, social isolation, physical distancing and the wearing of masks led to anxiety and depression in many people and created barriers to seeking and accessing support. It also had an impact on family functioning and how people went about meeting their needs. Weight gain owing to people not taking exercise during isolation was a real problem.

Perhaps the hardest part of having an MECC conversation is starting it, particularly in the time restraints of the job. These conversations, as that is what they are, are brief, use open questions and assist the person in making positive choices based on the best evidence (see Chapter 2). Furthermore, it should be a respectful conversation. The tone of an interaction is usually set by the way it is opened. What is actually said in greeting, or in opening a conversation, is of crucial importance, and tells each participant a great deal about how the other perceives their relationship and expects the interaction to proceed. A respectful conversation starts with the nurse asking the person's permission to hold a conversation. Asking permission to hold a conversation can help to build rapport, as well as creating trust and co-operation.

Examples of asking permission

- Do you mind if we talk about [insert behaviour]?
- Can we talk a bit about your [insert behaviour]?
- I noticed in your notes that you have hypertension. Do you mind if we talk about how different lifestyles affect hypertension?
- Would you like …?

- It sounds like … Can we explore …?
- Can I take a moment to run through what you said?

In holding an MECC conversation, we need to ask, advise and assist (NHS Midlands and East, 2012) (see Table 3.1). It is by *listening* to the person and what they have to say that we respond appropriately to their concerns. In *advising* the person, we give messages about the benefits of healthy lifestyle change and tips to achieve them. In *assisting* the person, we share information or signpost the person to where they can find local support.

Ask	Advise	Assist
You said you would like to give up smoking. Have you thought about how you might go about doing this?	Stopping smoking is the best thing you can do for your health. You're four times more likely to quit with help from an adviser compared to alone.	Your local well-being hub has information about local pharmacies and GP practices that provide stop smoking support. I can give you a leaflet, if you like? There are also useful tips and information about quitting on the One You and NHS Smokefree websites.

Table 3.1   Ask, advise, assist

However, if a contact is to truly count, the focus should be on the individual and their needs.

In structuring a conversation, we seek to empower the person to take ownership of their health. This is achieved by focusing on the individual's goals rather than what the professionals want to change and is actioned by developing a collaborative relationship between the nurse and the person. This involves helping people to assess where they are and what they would like to achieve, working collaboratively to help people plan how to achieve their goals and do things that they might have struggled with in the past, and challenging habits and beliefs that might have inhibited people or are barriers to positive change.

Case study: Astral

Astral is a 32-year-old woman who is being seen as an outpatient, who frequently misses her appointments, and at other times shows up without an appointment, often in crisis. She currently uses alcohol and tobacco and has started to use street drugs.

As you have developed a therapeutic relationship with Astral, you learn that she grew up in a household with a violent father who frequently assaulted her mother, her siblings and herself. Although now estranged from her father, the impact of his violence presents itself on a daily basis as Astral struggles to cope with the trauma she experienced.

Astral left school early, has few marketable skills and has never been able to hold a job for more than three months. Astral receives various state benefits which she claims are not enough to live on and often has no money come the end of the month to live on. Astral is currently in a relationship with a woman whom you suspect may be violent.

When we help others to consider and take various actions for themselves, it can help to examine – with them – some of the possible barriers that might impede their progress. It can be useful to do this before they actually take any action, so that they can be realistic in their expectations for success or not. Having a health-promoting conversation with Astral could prove difficult. While Astral leads a chaotic lifestyle, it maybe needs satisfying.

The idea behind an MECC conversation is not to tell the person what they should be doing but to raise the person's awareness of the problem behaviour and subsequently empowering the person to take action. The nurse does this by being a strong ally who encourages the person when needed. This is best achieved when we focus on the strengths and abilities of people to make lifestyle changes, focusing on the benefits of change and advising them as appropriate. This is largely done through active and reflective listening and challenging the person through the use of questioning, as well as affirming the client's freedom of choice and self-direction (see Chapter 2).

Concept summary: The WDEP system

When holding an MECC conversation the author uses what is referred to as the WDEP system. The WDEP system was developed by Robert Wubbolding (2011) and derives from Reality Therapy. It helps give structure to a conversation and puts the person at the centre of the problem-solving process, and is as follows:

W – What does the person want? (e.g. to lose weight)
D – What is the person doing? (e.g. eating unhealthy food; not taking exercise)
E – Evaluate. Is what the person is doing helping them to get what they want? Is it taking them in the direction they want to go? Is what they want achievable? Does it help the person to look at it in that way? How hard are they prepared to work at this? Is their current level of commitment working in their favour?
P – Plan. What plan does the person have for moving in their desired direction? Are they clear about what it is they will do? Is what they plan realistic? How will the person know when they have achieved it? How committed are they to doing it? Can they start doing it immediately?

The system offers individuals a way to discover what they want and to identify what they are doing to obtain or achieve what they want, and to evaluate their behaviour and plan to behave differently. The skill in using such a framework is to pitch these questions to the person in such a way that seeks to support their decision making and at the same time to motivate them.

Summarising an MECC conversation

When a lot of information has been exchanged, closure may be used by either party to summarise or clarify what has been covered and agreed on (see Chapter 2). Summaries are a special type of reflection where the nurse recaps what has occurred in all or part of an intervention or consultation. They can be used to start a conversation ('The last time we talked of you quitting smoking ...'), link points together ('So, you're saying that you're very busy at the moment and it would be difficult to commit to stopping smoking and taking up exercise ...') and end a conversation ('We're due to meet again in a week's time. I'll make sure to bring the literature I promised you on stopping smoking and go through that with you.').

Summaries communicate interest and understanding, as well as calling attention to important elements of the discussion. They may be used to shift attention or direction and prepare the patient to 'move on'. Summaries can highlight both sides of a patient's ambivalence about change, as well as promoting the development of discrepancy, by strategically selecting what information should be included and what can be minimised or excluded. Perhaps the greatest skill of holding an MECC conversation is knowing when to refer the person on to another professional or service. Activity 3.3 asks you to consider this in terms of where you are based.

Activity 3.3   Decision making

The final part of an MECC conversation is knowing when to refer a person to a particular service or not. Make a list of services within your local community that provide public health support. You may be surprised at the number you arrive at. Try to make time to visit some of these and learn more about what they have to offer. This will put you in a better position to help people. For example, Paul, one of the authors, has an interest in veteran mental health. There are a number of local charities and services where he lives in Norfolk that offer help and support to ex-servicemen and women with a mental illness, and that accept referrals outside of the NHS. The Walnut Tree Health and Well-being charity is one such service that has won national recognition (see **www.walnuttreehealthandwellbeing.co.uk**).

As local resources will differ from locality to locality, there is no outline answer at the end of the chapter.

MECC as an intervention

Health promotion interventions may be directed at a population or community, the systems that affect the health of those populations and/or individuals and their families. As an intervention, MECC is aimed at individuals and is based on the NICE (2007) behaviour change guidance, which defines behaviour change in four levels. MECC falls within levels 1 and 2 of these interventions.

Level 1 interventions consist of very brief interventions and the signposting of services, delivered whenever the opportunity arises in routine appointments and contacts. Very brief interventions take from 30 seconds to a couple of minutes. It enables the delivery of information to people or signposting them to sources of further help. It may also include other activities such as raising awareness of risks or providing encouragement and support for change.

Level 2 interventions consist of brief interventions, such as **motivational interviewing**, aimed at people whose health and well-being could be at risk (e.g. patients with high blood pressure who are overweight and at risk from a heart attack). This level of intervention uses brief intervention to hold a health/lifestyle conversation and may lead to referral for other interventions or more intensive support. An MECC conversation at this level can be broken down into three distinct parts:

1. asking individuals about their lifestyle and changes they may wish to make, when there is an appropriate opportunity to do so;

2. responding appropriately to the lifestyle issue(s) once raised;

3. taking the appropriate action to either give information, signpost or refer individuals to the support they need.

Level 3 interventions are extended brief interventions used by staff who regularly come into contact with people for 30 minutes or more (e.g. behavioural change programmes such as smoking cessation programmes) and are targeted in what they have to offer.

Level 4 interventions are expert or specialist interventions that are condition-specific or require additional specialist training, such as with people who are at higher risk of either illness or disease owing to such things as a compromised immune system (e.g. cancers of the immune system such as leukaemia, immune complex diseases).

It is important to note that in the literature there is no one clear definition of what constitutes brief advice, brief intervention and extended intervention. This creates a challenge in the interpretation and practical application of these interventions. It also highlights the need for the nurse to work within their limitations and you should only engage in conversations that you are happy holding. If you feel uncomfortable in the conversation, then this could be an indicator that you need to refer the person on or signpost them to a particular speciality or service. This again is an important part of the nurse's role and one that is sometimes neglected in clinical practice.

Hopefully, you have developed a sense that by holding even a very brief MECC conversation, you can have a positive impact on an individual's health and well-being. Healthcare is not just about providing for the sick and ill but recognising that it encompasses health-enhancing activities such as MECC. It is also about recognising that health promotion works on different levels and that nurses, as well as other healthcare professionals and workers, have an important role in promoting the health of others.

Chapter summary

MECC is about raising awareness of health and well-being and motivating people to make change. It can be considered a model of change intervention and provides a framework with which to guide health-promotion practice. The key message behind MECC is the same as the one running throughout this book: it is more effective to support and empower people to change than to enforce change on a person. When people come up with their own solutions, they are more likely to put them into action and maintain the changes that they make. However, it is important to remember that you are not responsible for the choices people make. In order to carry out a health-promotion intervention, nurses and other healthcare practitioners need to appreciate how health needs change over the lifespan, as well as incorporating this knowledge into our interventions with others in order to maximise the health and life chances of an individual. MECC is the responsibility of all those who work in health and social care.

Activities: Brief outline answers

Activity 3.1 Critical thinking (page 40)

People may be reluctant to talk about their health concerns because they:

- feel overwhelmed with the task of managing their health;
- have little confidence in their ability to have a positive impact on their health;
- misunderstand their role in the care process;
- have limited problem-solving skills;
- have had substantial experience of failing to manage their health and have become passive in managing their health;
- say that they would rather not think about their health.

Further reading

Nelson, A, de Normanville, C, Payne, K and Kelly, MP (2013) Making Every Contact Count: An Evaluation. *Public Health,* 127(7): 653–60.

This was the evaluation of the NHS Yorkshire and Humber competence framework, 'Prevention and Lifestyle Change', on which MECC is based.

Useful websites

www.makingeverycontactcount.co.uk

This website houses information on the MECC scheme and has a useful 'Linked Resources' section.

https://stpsupport.nice.org.uk/mecc/index.html

This page on the NICE website looks at the underpinning evidence base on which the MECC scheme is based.

www.gov.uk/government/publications/making-every-contact-count-mecc-practical-resources

These documents support the local implementation and evaluation of MECC activity and the development of training resources.

Chapter 4 Health promotion with individuals

NMC Future Nurse: Standards of Proficiency for Registered Nurses

This chapter will address the following platforms and proficiencies:

Platform 2: Promoting health and preventing ill health

At the point of registration, the registered nurse will be able to:

2.1 understand and apply the aims and principles of health promotion, protection and improvement and the prevention of ill health when engaging with people.

2.4 identify and use all appropriate opportunities, making reasonable adjustments when required, to discuss the impact of smoking, substance and alcohol use, sexual behaviours, diet and exercise on mental, physical and behavioural health and well-being, in the context of people's individual circumstances.

2.8 explain and demonstrate the use of up-to-date approaches to behaviour change to enable people to use their strengths and expertise and make informed choices when managing their own health and making lifestyle adjustments.

2.9 use appropriate communication skills and strength-based approaches to support and enable people to make informed choices about their care to manage health challenges in order to have satisfying and fulfilling lives within the limitations caused by reduced capability, ill health and disability.

2.10 provide information in accessible ways to help people understand and make decisions about their health, life choices, illness and care.

Chapter aims

After reading this chapter, you will be able to:

- describe the health promotion opportunities nurses have when caring for people;
- consider a social ecological view of health to support people with their health and well-being needs in a person-centred way;
- identify approaches that nurses can employ to empower people in self-management strategies.

Case study: Aled

Aled is a 24-year-old living in an inner-city area in Wales. He and his friends attend the local gym regularly.

I have been coming to this gym since leaving high school and have a small but close group of friends. We meet up at least three times a week to do bodybuilding together. I have really focused on developing my muscle mass and have a personal trainer. I am careful about what I eat and I take supplements to support my weight training. I get stressed if I haven't been to the gym for a couple of days.

I work full-time at a tech firm and I get involved with the interdepartmental sports activities. I have recently started a rugby team at work.

I took up bodybuilding as I was overweight as a child and I experienced years of bullying at school. I developed an eating disorder that resulted in me needing inpatient support at a specialist eating disorder unit. While I am better now, I still have body image issues, and this drives me to keep attending the gym.

I recently pulled a muscle when training and was not able to train for a few weeks. I started to feel low in mood, and this impacted on my eating patterns and emotional health. After one particularly bad day, I reverted to binge-eating unhealthy foods and afterwards felt the need to make myself vomit. It really scared me to think how quickly I had returned to the feelings I had as a child. Fortunately, I have a supportive family, and my mum encouraged me to go to the GP. The GP referred me to the counselling service to do a course of cognitive behavioural therapy (CBT), but there was a waiting list, so I hadn't started any sessions by the time I was fit enough to weight train again. Even so, I was able to speak to the practice nurse on a couple of occasions to work through some self-help strategies, which helped me feel more in control of my emotions and my thought processes. While I try to keep positive about my body image, the recent experience has made me realise that I am not as resilient as I thought I was, and I am hopeful that the CBT will help me to manage this in the future.

Introduction

The case study above demonstrates the complex nature of promoting health and well-being with individuals. On the surface, Aled is generally a fit and healthy young adult; however, his personal history has shaped his approach to his emotional and physical health. Whichever field of nursing we practise within, we need to understand the person's perceptions of health to be able to support them in meeting their health and well-being needs. Without this understanding, there is the potential that we apply a generic 'one-size-fits-all' version of health to people, which may not lead to positive and sustained health behaviours.

We work with people of all ages from diverse personal, social, economic and cultural backgrounds. This diversity provides us with a wealth of opportunities to develop and adapt our skills to promote health and well-being with a wide variety of people experiencing various health needs. We need to focus on effective and flexible communication strategies to provide person-centred care based on up-to-date knowledge and skills. This will enable us to share accurate health information with people and effectively utilise person-centred and goal-setting approaches to meet their health and well-being needs.

Some nurses have an additional Specialist Community Public Health Nursing (SCPHN) qualification, such as occupational health nurses, health visitors and school nurses. These nurses have a primary role in health promotion with individuals and groups from a specific sector of the population (NMC, 2021). Other nurses will have enhanced their practice with additional training (e.g. diabetes specialist nurses, sexual health nurses). Nevertheless, all nurses have a responsibility to promote health and well-being when working with people throughout their daily practice, as identified in standard 3.1 of *The Code: pay special attention to promoting well-being, preventing ill health and meeting the changing health and care needs of people during all life stages* (NMC, 2018b, page 7).

This chapter explores the importance of promoting health and well-being with people. We will consider the necessity of understanding the challenges facing people of all ages and with diverse circumstances to lead healthier lives and manage their health needs, as well as the strategies nurses can employ to empower them to attain their health goals.

Firstly, we will consider opportunities for promoting health and well-being in our daily practice. We will recap on the levels of interventions before considering how a social ecological perspective of health can help us to support people in a person-centred way. Finally, the chapter will consider extended brief and high-intensity interventions that can be effective in empowering people in self-management strategies.

Promoting health and well-being: interventions and opportunities

All health professionals promote health and well-being daily in a range of clinical settings, whether acute, community and primary healthcare or specialist health promotion services (e.g. smoking cessation, sexual health). We will mainly focus on nurses in this chapter, but it is important to recognise that promoting health and well-being involves multiprofessional working. Many people will engage with a range of professionals across many services to reach their health goals. Nurses will work collaboratively as part of a multiprofessional team with the person, and perhaps relevant significant others (such as parents or carers), to empower them to develop awareness and skills to manage their own health and well-being needs at a time and pace that is right for them. It is important to remember that respecting people's decisions to not engage in or to discontinue health promotion support is an essential factor in person-focused care. However, do bear in mind that when working with children, young people and vulnerable adults, you will need to be aware of safeguarding requirements in care provision. Where significant others such as parents and carers fail to meet their responsibilities to support the person with their health and well-being needs, this will involve exploration of the situation and escalation so that focused multi-agency working within legal safeguarding requirements can take place (HM Government 2018c, Care Act, 2014).

To recap our explorations in Chapter 3, we learned about 'very brief' or 'brief' interventions, where the principal aim is to engage the person in a short conversation about their health needs and potential risks to their health. Typically, these interventions involve identifying what the person knows about their health and well-being needs, as well as if they are interested in further advice and support.

In this chapter, we will focus on 'extended brief interventions' and 'high-intensity interventions'. These can be used when supporting people at various life stages and with diverse personal circumstances. In 'extended brief interventions', a more focused assessment of need and planning of interventions takes place for a series of sessions lasting up to 30 minutes each. Alternatively, 'high-intensity interventions' are those where the person requires a high level of focused support due to significant health needs, such as obesity, or a health condition that needs specialist advice, such as **chronic obstructive pulmonary disease** (COPD) (NICE, 2014a). These interventions are planned opportunities where the health professional provides focused health promotion with people who have sought support to improve their health and well-being, or where it is an element of their ongoing care (e.g. people with long-term conditions). Effective person-centred care will mean that nurses may also work with caregivers when planning effective interventions, depending on the person's specific needs and abilities. This is more likely with children and young people, and people with learning diabilities, but people with physical and psychological health needs may require caregiver support too.

The person may want to change a behaviour or make informed decisions and learn new skills to manage a condition that is impacting on their health and well-being. The nurse works with the person to explore their health needs, provide information to increase their knowledge so that they can make informed decisions, and develop planned activities with them to reach their health goals. These plans are tailored to best-practice approaches while taking into consideration the person's circumstances and harnessing their strengths.

There are many opportunities to promote health and well-being with people in our daily nursing practice. We work with people of all ages and abilities, so the types of 'extended brief interventions' will be diverse. For instance, children's nurses may engage with families and children in relation to healthy eating or physical and emotional well-being through play, tailored to both the developmental needs of the children and young people, and to the literacy needs of families and carers. Learning disability nurses may support people with learning disabilities to develop skills in managing their relationship and sexual health needs. Mental health nurses may work with people with mental health needs to self-manage their emotional well-being, including exploring the benefits of emotional well-being strategies such as walking and being in the natural environment. Adult nurses may support people to consider increasing their physical activity to support any weight-loss plans.

Some common health promotion opportunities aim to address health risks associated with people's health behaviours. Key **behavioural risk factors** are cigarette smoking, obesity, alcohol consumption (over the recommended 14 units per week), physical inactivity and consumption of less than five portions per day of fruit and vegetables. These risk factors are important as they impact on people's health and quality of life, as well as resulting in conditions that are largely preventable such as cardiovascular disease, diabetes, high cholesterol, hypertension and chronic pain (NHS Digital, 2018a). Importantly, the 2018 *Health Survey for England* (NHS Digital, 2018a) identified that while only 36 per cent of the population had one risk factor, over 54 per cent of men and 47 per cent of women had two or more risk factors, which increases their risk of developing one or more health conditions as a result of their health behaviours. It is important to be aware that people who have developed health conditions as a result of their health behaviours have not only physical needs, but there is a further impact on their social and economic status. Adults may not be able to work or have limited means to access social activities for them and their family, which can negatively impact on emotional well-being. People of all ages and backgrounds are influenced by social determinants such as the environment they live in, social and cultural networks, education and employment, therefore health behaviours cannot be taken in isolation when providing services (Marmot et al., 2020).

Health conditions linked to behavioural risk factors also have an impact on the health service and the health economy, as resources are diverted to treat these conditions that could be used more effectively in preventative healthcare. There is a significant cost to the health service and the wider economy. You may be aware of healthcare trusts purchasing bariatric equipment to be able to care effectively for people who are obese. A report by Holmes (2021) identified that obesity across the lifespan is a significant health concern, with rates of individuals either overweight or obese leading to increased hospital admissions due to obesity-related disorders. While obesity at any age is of concern, obesity in children can have a lifelong impact on the person's health and well-being if not addressed during childhood. These impacts include increased risk of heart disease, some cancers, musculoskeletal problems and a negative impact on emotional well-being. Rates of obesity have risen highest in deprived communities, leading to poorer health outcomes for those who are most at risk in our society. If person-focused preventative measures can be implemented successfully, this will have a beneficial impact for people and health services. Therefore, local and national health policies focus on raising awareness of health behaviours for people across the lifespan, not only to prevent ill health, but to support people who are already engaging in unhealthy activities in reducing and stopping unhealthy behaviours.

Supporting people with their health and well-being needs requires us to have an awareness of their circumstances and personal and social resources to enable provision of effective person-centred care.

Concept summary: Person-centred care

Person-centred care refers to a process that is people focused, promotes independence and autonomy, provides choice and control and is based on a collaborative team philosophy. It takes into account people's needs and views and builds relationships with family members. It recognises that care should be holistic and so includes a spiritual, pastoral and religious dimension. The delivery of person-centred care requires both safe and effective care and should result in a good experience for people.

(NHS Wales, 2019)

Person-centred care focuses on the needs of the person rather than the needs of the health professional, healthcare organisation or health system. The engagement of people in influencing and taking control of their own health needs is central to this approach. A key element of person-centred care in health promotion is developing an understanding of the perspective of the individual in order to meet their needs.

A social ecological perspective of health and well-being

A report in 2018 identified that diseases such as heart disease, some cancers, cardiovascular disease and COPD were consistently the most significant causes of mortality and morbidity in adults in the UK across both genders (Steel et al., 2018). While the **SARS-CoV-2** virus will have impacted on the causes of morbidity and mortality across the population since February 2020, it is important to be aware that the diseases highlighted in Steele et al.'s (2018) report have not lessened and continue to impact on the health of adults in the UK (PHE 2021a). Awareness of causes of morbidity and mortality are important when we are working with people so that we take a broad view of influencing factors in the wider environment that may be impacting on their personal circumstances. Taking a social ecological approach can assist us in exploring with people the different factors influencing their health and health choices.

An ecological perspective was introduced by Urie Bronfenbrenner in 1979 in his theory that focused on an ecological view of child development (Bronfenbrenner, 2005). Since Bronfenbrenner's early work, the **social ecological model** has been developed and expanded within health and social care (Rayner and Lang, 2012). It is particularly useful in conceptualising factors that influence people's health and well-being when we are providing interventions. The social ecological perspective is commonly applied to public health policies, which we will explore further in Chapter 7.

Figure 4.1 provides a visual representation of the social ecological model and the various elements that interact and influence individuals throughout their lives.

As nurses we are adept at considering the person as a whole rather than focusing solely on their health needs, and the social ecological model supports a more

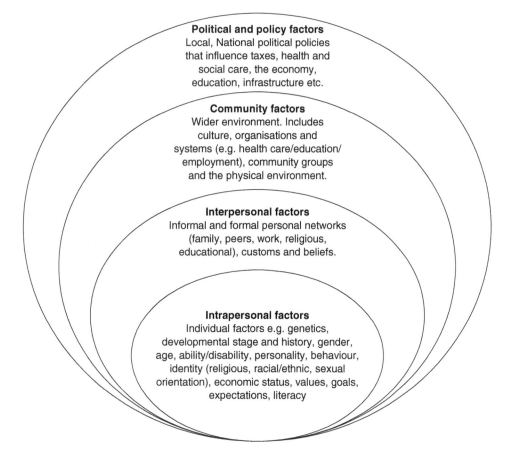

Figure 4.1 The social ecological model (adapted from Bronfenbrenner, 2005; Rayner and Lang, 2012)

(Author's own diagram adapted from information within Bronfenbrenner 2005, and Rayner and Lang 2012)

in-depth approach to exploring people's circumstances, identifying what life experiences have had an influence on them, and what aspects are currently impacting on their health and well-being. As you can see, it is not only the biological and intrapersonal factors that impact on the person, but also social, economic, environmental and political factors. These factors dynamically interact to influence how individuals will understand and experience their world, dependent on the opportunities and limitations they have experienced in the past and are currently experiencing. Understanding the factors that are influencing people will enable you to gain an insight into what resources they have (whether personal, social or material), which can be activated to support them in managing their health needs. Importantly, this approach may also enable you to see what limitations exist (again whether personal, social or material), which would need to be considered to ensure any interventions or expectations are realistic and achievable, and where additional support or services may be needed.

To further help us understand how a social ecological approach can provide a greater understanding of people in our care, we can consider the potential influences on people during their lifespan. Key life stages are pre-conception, infancy and early years, childhood and adolescence, working age and adult, and older adult (see Figure 4.2). A **life course** approach is a key theme within *Future Nurse: Standards of Proficiency for Registered Nurses* (NMC, 2018a).

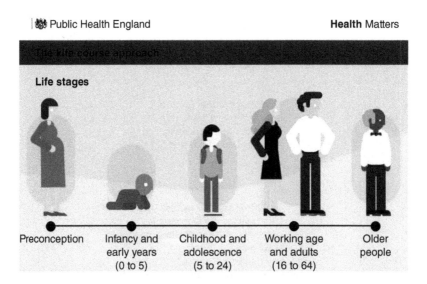

Figure 4.2 The life course approach (PHE, 2019b)

To support you to gain insight into these approaches, Activity 4.1 uses both the social ecological model and a life course approach to enable you to consider how your health and well-being has been influenced by various factors during your lifespan.

Activity 4.1   Reflection

Using the social ecological model and a life course approach, consider the influences on you as you have developed throughout your life. You may find it helpful to draw a time-line and indicate on it where certain key points in your life have had an influence, before reflecting on what this means in terms of your own health and well-being.

Consider:

- elements that affected you during your life stages (e.g. health – physical and emotional – educational and social elements);
- elements of your family and culture/religion that have influenced your choices and decisions relating to your health, health behaviours and lifestyle (e.g. diet/exercise, social activities);
- the community aspects that have influenced you (e.g. the environment you live in/ have lived in, your schooling);
- the wider influences on your current circumstances (e.g. political, educational, economic policies).

What are the key stages of your development and the wider influences that have had an impact on your health and well-being? Are there any elements that have had a significant impact on your health? Do you think that any of these elements influence your personal approach to your health and well-being now?

As this is a personal reflection, there is no outline answer at the end of the chapter.

Hopefully, this exploration of your life history will have helped you to gain an insight into how important background information is when supporting people with their health needs. You can do this activity with other members of your family, such as parents and grandparents, to gain an insight into the differing experiences within your own close interpersonal network.

Considerations of the various social ecological factors when providing person-centred care can support effective provision of services; this is particularly helpful when supporting people with complex holistic care needs, as highlighted in the case study below.

Case study: Ahmed

Ahmed is a ten-year-old refugee from Syria.

I live in supported accommodation for refugees with my mother and older sister in an inner-city area in the UK. I witnessed the fighting in Syria first hand when my father was killed, and I feel

(Continued)

(Continued)

very sad that he died. I was severely injured by shrapnel and had to have my left leg amputated below the knee. Since coming to the UK, I have met many people when having my treatment. I am learning to walk again with help from a physiotherapist, and I am meeting weekly with a psychologist as I am having flashbacks to when my father died. They tell me I have something called post-traumatic stress, which is affecting my sleeping, and I keep feeling very frightened at noises and banging. I have just started to go to a school, which I am enjoying. I am learning new English words every day and I have met some new friends. My mother and I are meeting a nurse today in school because he can help me and my teachers look at ways I can settle into school.

The social ecological model can help us to begin to think about Ahmed's circumstances, as well as what elements may require our care and support. Activity 4.2 now asks you to explore this further.

Activity 4.2   Critical thinking

You are on placement with the school nurse, Jake, who has been asked to support Ahmed and the teaching staff with managing his health needs in school. Before you go into the school to meet with Ahmed, his mother and his teachers, Jake discusses Ahmed's history with you to identify what may be the key elements that he will need to be mindful of.

Using the case study information, the social ecological model and your knowledge of life stages:

- What do you think are the factors that *have* affected Ahmed's health and well-being before he arrived in the UK?
- What do you think are the factors that *are currently* affecting Ahmed's health and well-being?
- What do you think are the factors that *will potentially* affect Ahmed's health and well-being in the future?

An outline answer is provided at the end of the chapter.

It is clear from the case study and from your likely responses to Activity 4.2 that to provide effective person-centred care and promote health and well-being with Ahmed and his family, consideration needs to be given to:

- effective communication (potentially using translation services);
- his immediate health needs (both physical and emotional);
- developing social networks and continuing his education;
- consideration of longer-term health needs and goals.

From a health promotion perspective, engagement with Ahmed, his mother and teachers may focus on how he can access his education while recovering and adapting to the loss of a limb. This can include what he needs to support him in mobilising around school and accessing his lessons, where he can go if he is feeling emotionally overwhelmed, and who he can talk to. Engaging Ahmed in his care is important, even though he is a young person. His wishes and feelings should feature in all plans that are devised so that he can develop skills in self-management from an early stage.

Developing a positive health promotion relationship with people

Interventions to support people to manage their health and well-being have a strong ethos of person-centred approaches because evidence has shown that this approach results in sustained self-management and better outcomes for people.

Research summary: Patient activation

People may not engage in behaviour change or manage their health due to limited knowledge, low levels of literacy to be able to process health information, low confidence in their abilities and a history of failing in previous attempts to improve their health and well-being.

Hibbard and Gilburt (2014) wrote a report for the King's Fund that looked at the concept of 'patient activation'. Patient activation is defined as the *knowledge, skills and confidence a person has in managing their own healthcare* (Hibbard and Gilburt, 2014, page 3). While this is especially important in terms of people living with long-term conditions, it is equally applicable for all individuals.

The authors identified that increased levels of activation improve the person's ability to manage and maintain their health. However, low activation increases the person's use of healthcare services (e.g. emergency services). Repeated readmissions are costly to not only the person, but also to the health service and provision of services. It is difficult for providers to develop preventative services when funding is needed to care for people needing recurrent inpatient services.

Patient activation incorporates both behavioural and motivational elements. Key to the concept is that people need to feel able to not only understand and master new skills but have the confidence and motivation to carry out and maintain the skills and activities to manage their own health needs.

If we return to the opening case study of this chapter, we can apply patient activation elements to Aled's situation. Aled has high levels of motivation and skills to manage his approach to his previous eating disorder. He has developed and adapted both behavioural and motivational actions to self-manage his physical and mental health needs. Even though he had a relapse in his mental health, he was able to source support effectively to enable him to manage his health in the short term. He is willing and able to engage in cognitive behavioural therapy (CBT), which will enable him to continue to self-manage his health needs in the future.

Engaging effectively with people

As you will have read in Chapter 2, the way we communicate with people is very important in promoting health and well-being. While a brief intervention conversation supports people in starting to think about their health needs, interventions requiring more frequent and intensive interactions require the healthcare practitioner to develop enhanced skills and have the ability to use a wider range of resources.

Therefore, nurses need to develop a range of skills, from general to specialist approaches depending on the type and intensity of the intervention and the needs of the person engaging in services. Depending on the role of the nurse, the local service provision and the type of intervention, approaches can include motivational interviewing techniques, CBT, solution-focused therapy, stress management (e.g. mindfulness techniques) and self-management education. Sometimes this will be delivered by the health professional (depending on their role and their skill set), but referral to another service may be necessary.

Health coaching has been recommended as an approach to the delivery of health promotion interventions. Evidence suggests that health coaching can be useful in a range of health interventions, including behaviour change, as well as helping people who have long-term conditions to manage their health needs (Edwards et al., 2018). Health coaching changes the dynamic of the health promotion relationship to one that promotes people as active participants in their care. Training health professionals in health coaching techniques enables the health intervention to be a more effective interaction.

Health coaching aims to be person-centred, empowering, focused and collaborative. A key strength of the health coaching approach is the flexibility for the health professional to use a variety of techniques to enhance the interaction with the person, whatever their age or cognitive ability, although you may need to engage with carers depending on the age and cognitive ability of the person. These include developing core communication strategies further and moving away from advice-giving approaches to feeling comfortable with active listening, silence and reflecting with the person about their perceptions of their health needs. The person is encouraged to identify their own areas of need and explore barriers to change in order to set their own goals. Health coaching is a way of working with people rather than a specific set of tools. Understanding patient activation, motivation, people's approaches to learning about their health and their readiness for change are all elements needed to provide effective support.

Engaging in effective behaviour change

As we explored in Chapter 1, healthcare professionals can utilise behaviour change models when planning health promotion interventions with people. Many resources and guidance documents focus on behaviour change approaches when supporting people to manage their health and well-being effectively. National guidance documents are helpful in assisting us to ensure that our approaches are person-centred and are underpinned by evidence-based practice. You can search on the national guidance websites, such as the National Institute for Health and Care Excellence (NICE) or the Scottish Intercollegiate Guidelines Network (SIGN), for up-to-date guidance on a broad range of health topics, including behaviour change best practice approaches.

In engaging people in behaviour change conversations, NICE recommends that practitioners assess the person's needs, including physical, mental, socio-economic and environmental elements, in order to effectively plan interventions (NICE, 2014a). Health promotion interventions should also encompass best practice approaches that support people in developing the knowledge, skills and abilities to feel able to make positive changes to their lives. This will include an increased awareness of factors that influence their behaviours and the potential actions they can take.

People are more receptive to change when there are trigger events that raise their awareness (PHE, 2020a). These could be: national events such as the annual no smoking day; someone they know being diagnosed with a health condition such as type 2 diabetes, COPD, heart disease or cancer; or their own health condition prompting them to address an aspect of their health (e.g. losing weight to be eligible for hip replacement surgery).

Let's consider how working with people can improve their knowledge and self-care abilities.

Scenario part 1: Emilia – initial brief intervention

You are on placement with the general practice nurse in a GP surgery based in a remote rural community. Emilia is 40 years old and identifies her ethnicity as Black British. She has been invited to attend a well-being appointment as part of the NHS Health Check provision (NHS, 2019). Emilia's height and weight are recorded; her BMI is 28 kg/m² and her waist circumference is 87 cm.

As we will explore in Activity 4.3, understanding these clinical measurements will guide the potential health promotion activity.

Activity 4.3   Critical thinking and evidence-based practice

Consider Emilia's baseline measurements.

What do you need to know in order to interpret these measurements? What do the measurements tell you? Which national guidance sources can be used to support best practice?

An outline answer is provided at the end of the chapter.

This activity enabled you to consider your knowledge and locate key guidance to support your clinical practice and enable you to assess what support Emilia may need. As highlighted in Chapter 3, the initial brief intervention conversation is vitally important to ascertain if the person is willing and able to engage in any interventions. Developing your communication skills to promote kind, caring, empathic and compassionate approaches with people in your care is essential.

In this scenario, establishing a good rapport with Emilia will enable the nurse to ascertain her views of her weight, as she may not consider it a problem. It is important not to assume that Emilia has not tried to lose weight before, as she may already be engaging in self-managed weight-loss programmes and be happy with her current weight-loss progress.

West and Michie (2020) identify in the COM-B (Capability, Opportunities, Motivation – Behaviour) model that there are three main components which interact to influence behaviours:

1. Capability (the knowledge and skills of the individual);
2. Opportunity (the external factors that enable the behaviour change); and/or
3. Motivation (the way individuals view and engage/disengage with the behaviour).

A person's capability and opportunity will influence their motivation to engage in the behaviour. In this scenario, the nurse aims to ascertain whether Emilia is aware that she is overweight, whether she has tried to lose weight recently and if she would like to consider approaches to support her in doing so. It is important to be mindful of whether Emilia has any deficits in health literacy or a cognitive impairment which will impact on the interaction and any subsequent interventions. Emilia may also have an emotional response to being asked about her weight (e.g. defensive, anger, distress, a more positive response), and there may be deep-seated psychological elements to how Emilia engages with food and her body image. Therefore, sensitive questioning is vital to engage her in further conversations. Using the capability/opportunity/motivation approach can enable the nurse to assess whether Emilia is receptive to change, as well as what personal, physical and social resources she may have to engage in the interventions.

> ## Scenario part 2: Emilia – extended brief intervention
>
> Emilia has asked for support to reduce her weight. The assessment process identified that she does not have any multi-morbidities such as type 2 diabetes or hypertension or any deficits in her health literacy. NICE guidance recommends both diet and exercise advice for people who are overweight (NICE, 2014b); therefore, a plan is required to enable effective diet and exercise goals.
>
> When assessing Emilia's circumstances, she says she had been thinking about trying to lose weight for a while but did not know where to start. Her family had been talking about it recently as her children had been doing healthy eating lessons at school. She does not do regular exercise, but she enjoys walking. She works every day as a receptionist, and when she gets home she often chooses something that is quick to do for tea, such as chips and pizza or ready meals. Emilia and her husband drink less than five units of alcohol per week. Emilia suggests that snacking is her biggest challenge. She likes crisps as a snack, and she says she eats approximately three to four packets a day. Neither she nor her family have any food allergies and they like most things. When exploring alternatives to crisps, Emilia says she especially likes yoghurt and apples. She has a group of friends who live in her local village, and she thinks they may help her to achieve her health goals.

Goal setting

As we have seen, people who are active partners in their care are more likely to effectively manage and maintain their health and well-being. A key element is the effective setting of realistic goals. NICE (2014a) recommends that goals are developed by the person with support from the health professional, as well as factoring in the potential for the person to relapse during the behaviour change process. These allow the person to establish their own effective 'if/then' coping strategies (e.g. 'If this happens, then I will do …'). This reflects the evidence base on behaviour change, which recognises that individuals are likely to experience challenges and relapse in their journey to achieving their goals (Prochaska and DiClemente, 1983), and therefore goals need to factor in these events to support and sustain behaviour change. There is also further evidence that identifying with the person whether they have a personal or social support network may be beneficial in motivating them with their behaviour change activities (West and Michie, 2020).

We can use the mnemonic SMART to assist us when setting goals with individuals:

- Specific: The goal is clear and focused.
- Measurable: The goal has a defined outcome.

- Agreed with the individual: The individual is in control of the goal.
- Realistic: The goal is manageable (this requires a good understanding of the person's needs).
- Time-bound: There is a timescale applied to the goal (which is also realistic in itself).

Using the SMART goal-setting approach, Activity 4.4 gives you the opportunity to develop some simple goals for Emilia.

Activity 4.4 Critical thinking

Devise two *simple* SMART goals based on the information provided by Emilia in part 2 of the scenario, one based on her snack intake (diet) and one based on exercise.

What will be the 'if/then' action for each goal? Who else can support Emilia in achieving the goals she sets?

An outline answer is provided at the end of the chapter.

Hopefully, you were able to consider some simple initial goals to support Emilia's health behaviour change. It is important that people remain motivated and are supported through the ups and downs of the behaviour change journey. Therefore, developing a strong healthcare relationship will assist greater understanding of the practical and personal (including emotional) elements that influence people's behaviours.

As goals are reached, new goals are set that are more challenging but continue to be within the person's abilities as they will dictate the development of their goals. Support, encouragement and motivation increase the person's self-belief and ability to manage their own health needs and challenges in the future, so that eventually Health Professional support is reduced or ceases altogether. Of course, if Emilia had any additional needs such as physical health co-morbidities, a cognitive impairment and/or a psychological disorder, as nurses we would need to ensure Emilia's additional needs are accounted for within the planned intervention. This may require smaller goals, planning a longer time to achieve them, or goals that consider best practice guidelines related to a particular health condition.

The ultimate goal of any health promotion intervention is for people to self-manage and sustain their health and well-being needs, either independently or with the help of caregivers as necessary. When people are empowered to self-manage, they use health services more effectively, which increases their coping strategies (National Voices, 2014). Healthcare providers can then target services where they are needed the most.

Chapter summary

This chapter has introduced you to the various elements we can consider when working with people to improve their health and well-being, including consideration of social ecological factors. Health promoting activities are important to not only enable people to live well for longer, but also take control to manage their own health and well-being. Health promotion can occur in a variety of situations and at various levels of intensity depending on the needs of the person. Central to this approach is the importance of the person being empowered to actively engage in their own health management. Key to any health promotion intervention is enabling people to increase control over their health and well-being through the setting of realistic and achievable goals.

Ultimately, there are benefits to both people and the health service in empowering people to manage their own health and well-being needs.

Activities: Brief outline answers

Activity 4.2   Critical thinking (page 56)

While there may be many elements that affect Ahmed, here are a few to consider when supporting his care and promoting his health and well-being. We have intentionally not indicated whether any of these elements are positive or negative, as it would be important to seek Ahmed's views on this.

The factors that *have* affected his health and well-being are:

- fleeing his home country where there is a conflict;
- witnessing fighting and the death of his father;
- remaining with his mother and sister;
- receiving a life-changing injury, needing emergency care.

The factors that *are* affecting his health and well-being are:

- post-traumatic stress and bereavement;
- recovering from a lower limb amputation;
- being in a new country, meeting new people and having limited (but improving) understanding of the language;
- living with his mother and sister in supported accommodation;
- attending school;
- receiving multi-agency support.

The factors that *will potentially* affect his health and well-being are:

- Ahmed is ten (life stage: adolescence);
- Ahmed has had a lower limb amputation, and he is learning to walk again and may need further surgery;
- Ahmed is learning English at school, and his ability to understand and engage in his care will likely improve over time;
- Ahmed's recovery from post-traumatic stress and his amputation may have an ongoing impact on his emotional and mental well-being during his life.

Activity 4.3   Critical thinking and evidence-based practice (page 60)

Emilia's measurements show that she is overweight. Her waist circumference is high, and this indicates that she is at greater risk of health conditions associated with her weight. There is potential to explore diet and exercise interventions with her. The initial conversation will consider Emilia's opinion of her weight and if she feels she is ready for support. Health professionals can use the NICE guidelines (NICE, 2014b) as a basis for identifying and managing health-promotion activities with people who are overweight or obese.

Activity 4.4   Critical thinking (page 62)

Diet: The initial aim is to reduce Emilia's daily intake of high-calorie snacks and replace them with lower-calorie snacks. Other diet activities would include exploring with Emilia her approach to meal planning and her food and drink choices, and when shopping is managed within the family.

Goal: Emilia will reduce her intake of crisps to one packet per day for the next seven days, replacing them with an apple or a pot of low-fat, low-sugar yoghurt. If Emilia is unable to reduce to one packet of crisps per day, then she will try to reduce it to two packets for three days and then reduce to one packet each day after that.

Support: Emilia's family may be able to support her to reduce her snack intake by joining in with consuming healthier snacks. This may influence the amount of crisps the family needs/intends to buy.

Exercise: The aim is to increase Emilia's physical activity. NICE guidance recommends that people should engage in moderate-intensity exercise for 30 minutes at least five days per week, but to prevent obesity this should increase to 45–60 minutes per day (NICE, 2014b). As Emilia doesn't currently exercise, there will need to be a gradual increase in her activity levels.

Goal: Emilia will go for a 30-minute walk three times in the next seven days. If she is not able to manage 30 minutes, then she will walk for 20 minutes.

Support: Exercise can be a social event, so Emilia could go for a walk with her family or friends.

Useful websites

https://assets.publishing.service.gov.uk/government/uploads/system/uploads/attachment_data/file/769489/MECC_Training_quality_marker_checklist_updates.pdf

Public Health England has produced several resources on MECC which you may like to explore further. This resource has helpful links to information related to key health targets.

www.e-lfh.org.uk/programmes/all-our-health/

Health Education England has developed 'All Our Health' training resources which are helpful in developing your understanding of a range of health and well-being topics.

www.nice.org.uk

www.sign.ac.uk

Both the National Institute for Health and Care Excellence (NICE) and the Scottish Intercollegiate Guidelines Network (SIGN) are important websites to locate national guidance and advice relating to health and social care topics.

Chapter 5 Health promotion and the family

NMC Future Nurse: Standards of Proficiency for Registered Nurses

This chapter will address the following platforms and proficiencies:

Platform 2: Promoting health and preventing ill health

At the point of registration, the registered nurse will be able to:

2.1   understand and apply the aims and principles of health promotion, protection and improvement and the prevention of ill health when engaging with people.

2.5   promote and improve mental, physical, behavioural and other health-related outcomes by understanding and explaining the principles, practice and evidence base for health screening programmes.

2.6   understand the importance of early years and childhood experiences and the possible impact on life choices, mental, physical and behavioural health and well-being.

2.7   understand and explain the contribution of social influences, health literacy, individual circumstances, behaviours and lifestyle choices to mental, physical and behavioural health outcomes.

2.11 promote health and prevent ill health by understanding and explaining to people the principles of pathogenesis, immunology and the evidence base for immunisation, vaccination and herd immunity.

Chapter aims

After reading this chapter, you will be able to:

- discuss the influence families have on the health and well-being of their family members, including the importance of disease prevention;
- consider the impact of people's **health literacy** in enabling effective health education with people and families;
- discuss the importance of supporting families to develop coping and resilience strategies to manage the health and well-being needs of their members.

Case study: Rosie

Rosie is 24 years old and lives in Wales. Rosie's birth was difficult and she became hypoxic during the delivery. After close monitoring in early childhood, Rosie was diagnosed with spastic cerebral palsy, affecting her upper limbs and speech. She has some problems with fine motor movements in her hands and does exercises to improve her dexterity. She also has mild learning difficulties. Rosie receives support from a speech therapist and has regular physiotherapy. Rosie wears braces on her arms to support her movements and takes various medications to manage pain and discomfort. When she was 13 years old, Rosie was diagnosed with anxiety, which is exacerbated in social situations as people can say unkind things to her and her parents, or stare.

Rosie is transitioning to Adult Services now that she is nearing her 25th birthday, and she has made the decision to move into supported living accommodation.

I know Mum is feeling upset about my decision to move to my new flat. Mum and Dad have been there all the way for me; through those early days after my birth when she said she felt so much guilt and fear, during the nights when I was in so much pain I cried myself to sleep in Mum's arms, and I will never forget the joy on Dad's face when, despite my learning difficulty, I got 8 out of 10 in my spelling test at school. They have had to make so many decisions for me about my care, and Mum stopped work for a while so she could be there for me and take me to all my appointments. It will be strange not being back at home all the time, and I will miss our late-night chats. Mind you, my support worker is setting up my flat with the internet so I can video-chat with them any time I want. I will still need them, though, to help me with the things I still find tricky. Although my support worker will help me with the day-to-day things like filling in forms or paying bills, when it comes to decisions about my care needs, I will still check with Mum and Dad first.

Introduction

The above case study demonstrates that while Rosie is a young adult and able to make most of her own decisions, her relationship with her parents significantly contributes to the management of her health and well-being. This is because her family have played an important part in her development and life choices throughout her childhood and into early adulthood.

Promoting health and well-being with people will inevitably involve family members and key caregivers. As we have seen in Chapter 4, health promotion does not occur in a vacuum focused solely on the person. People are influenced by their interpersonal network throughout their lives, and therefore it is vital that nurses can work effectively with people and their families or caregivers to support health and well-being needs. Nurses need to understand family dynamics and customs when providing healthcare services, as well as strengthening families to cope with health needs and related decision making.

Continuing on from Chapter 4, this chapter will take a life course perspective to consider the ways that families influence the health and well-being of individual members, as well as the role families play in disease prevention. We will explore health education perspectives, including the importance of understanding health literacy in ensuring health promotion interventions meet people's needs. Finally, we will consider the importance of strengthening resilience and **coping strategies** within families when addressing health and well-being needs.

For the purposes of this chapter, 'family' is defined as those related to the person biologically or by law, or closely cohabiting with them within a personal relationship.

Health education and health literacy

In order to engage effectively to manage health and well-being needs, people need to be able to navigate services, develop an understanding of their health needs and learn new skills.

Health education is an integral component of interventions that promote health and well-being with people (Whitehead, 2018). It is an essential element of wider health promotion approaches that includes strategic and political drivers within national policies that consider individual, community and population health. Working with people, families and groups in a sustained way to empower and develop skills and behaviours to promote health and well-being is the main premise of health education.

In health education, the mode of delivery of the health education activity will require the nurse to be aware of a wide range of factors relating to the person and their family. A skill may require manual dexterity or physical stamina. Learning about a health condition and the interventions required will involve communication and mental processing skills. It is a legal requirement to provide accessible information to people with disabilities and impairments who use health and social care services (NHS England, 2017). However, the Health Education England health literacy resource identifies that the average reading age of adults in England is 11–14 years old (HEE, 2017). This is an important factor to understand when providing health education in a variety of mediums and so we should also ensure we consider the level of health literacy of all people who use services. There will often be an element of written information within a health education interaction to support verbal and visual learning, so the way in which information is presented and the literacy ability of the people accessing it are important considerations. This may be particularly relevant if you are a Children and Young People nurse, or a Learning Disability nurse, although all Adult nurses and Mental Health nurses working with people across the lifespan with physical, mental and cognitive impairments need to be aware too. Ensuring that we have an awareness of the attributes and challenges in terms of the learning needs of the people within a family is an essential element of successful health education. Activity 5.1 requires you to reflect on your experiences in practice within your particular field of nursing.

Activity 5.1   Reflection

From your field-specific clinical practice experiences, what different activities can you identify where people and family members engaged in health education relating to a health condition, or were taught a particular skill? What individual and family elements did you and the nurse need to take into consideration when preparing for the intervention? What challenges did you and the nurse face when working with the person or their family? What approaches did you and the nurse use to educate the person and their family?

An outline answer is provided at the end of the chapter.

Hopefully, this activity has highlighted that we engage in activities to educate people about their health needs on a daily basis, so you may have identified numerous examples when you observed, or participated in, a health education intervention. No doubt, some of these interventions may have been difficult and the nurse may have felt that there were significant obstacles interfering with a successful intervention. As we explored in Chapter 4, empowering, person-centred approaches will motivate individuals and result in sustained change, and there are many elements to consider that impact on people's engagement with the intervention. One key element to a successful intervention is the health literacy of individuals and family members. This is especially important where family members are primary caregivers, such as parents of children and young people, or carers for people with learning disabilities or cognitive impairments.

Concept summary: Health literacy

Health literacy has been defined as the cognitive and social skills which determine the motivation and ability of individuals to gain access to, understand and use information in ways which promote and maintain good health. Health literacy means more than being able to read pamphlets and successfully make appointments. By improving people's access to health information and their capacity to use it effectively, health literacy is critical to empowerment.

Defined this way, health literacy goes beyond a narrow concept of health education and individual behaviour-oriented communication, and addresses the environmental, political and social factors that determine health. Health education, in this more comprehensive understanding, aims to influence not only individual lifestyle decisions, but also raises awareness of the determinants of health, and encourages individual and collective actions which may lead to a modification of these determinants.

(WHO, 2009)

The NHS Digital Service Manual (2021) clarifies that people who have low levels of health literacy are less able to understand health information and to confidently engage with healthcare resources, and this includes being able to navigate health systems successfully. People may have low health literacy because of learning difficulties, deficits in their general education due to either non-engagement or a specified learning need, or they may have a new health condition that has impaired their cognitive function. People who are new to the UK, such as international workers or refugees, may also be unfamiliar with our health services and there may be language barriers; therefore, the medium in which we are communicating to people will need to be modified accordingly.

Assessing the health literacy of the people you are engaging with can be difficult. People may appear to show understanding but then be unable to sustain management of the skill or retain the information. Modifying our communication approach can be beneficial in checking people's understanding to support effective health promotion.

'Teach back' and 'chunk and check'

Two simple yet effective techniques are 'teach back' and 'chunk and check'. They can be used together to enable a more effective and empowering interaction (The Health Literacy Place, 2022).

In 'teach back', you ask the person to tell you in their own words what they have heard and understood about the instruction, the information you have given them, or the skill you have demonstrated. Not only does this allow the person to be engaged in the interaction, but it provides you with the opportunity to reinforce or amend (rather than correct) their understanding and, if relevant, the demonstration of the skill. In 'chunk and check', information is separated into manageable chunks and the person's understanding of the information is then checked. We can explore a health promotion opportunity by reconnecting with Rosie from the opening case study.

Scenario: Rosie's health appointment

Rosie has been to her local doctor's surgery for her first smear test. She is talking to the nurse about using condoms with her new partner, Elliot. Rosie asks if the nurse would show her how to put on a condom properly to minimise the risk of sexually transmitted infection. The nurse uses a condom demonstrator, condoms and an easy-to-read information leaflet. Rosie has the opportunity to practise using the equipment.

Activity 5.2 explores how we can use simple techniques to undertake an effective health promotion intervention with Rosie.

Activity 5.2   Critical thinking and communication

Imagine you are the nurse working with Rosie providing education and support to enable her to use condoms effectively. What aspects do you need to consider in terms of Rosie's health literacy and understanding? Describe how you would use 'teach back' and 'chunk and check' methods. What could you do to make the session even more effective?

An outline answer is available at the end of the chapter.

This activity is intended to highlight some simple skills you can utilise within health interventions. The 'chunk and check' and 'teach back' methods can be replicated in numerous health education activities so we would encourage you to consider examples of how you can utilise this approach within different scenarios relating to your own field of practice.

It is very positive that Rosie is keen to protect herself and her partner during sexual intercourse. Her engagement also demonstrates a level of health literacy in that she is able to navigate the health service provision and understand the importance of disease prevention in relation to her own health and well-being needs.

People with lower health literacy may not be able to articulate their needs for a range of reasons and so part of our role as nurses is to be aware of factors that may influence accessibility. In addition to a person-centred approach, it is helpful to be aware of the profile of the local population so that we can recognise potential gaps in provision and ensure services are accessible. This may include being mindful of the opportunities that impact people and their families in the local community, such as education opportunities, levels of socio-economic deprivation and the demographics of the population.

The family contribution to health and well-being

In this next section we take a life course perspective to visualise the contribution of families to the health and well-being of their members. As we progess through this section, do take time to reflect on people and their families who you may have already cared for in your field of nursing to consider their life perspectives.

Pre-conception, infancy and early years, and child and adolescent life stages

Parents play a vital role in their children's health pre-birth and throughout childhood. They have an essential role in the physical and emotional well-being of their children, in disease prevention and in supporting their children to develop the social skills necessary to communicate within their social networks. Some parents are not able to care for their children for various reasons, such as relationship breakdown, mental or physical ill health, safeguarding concerns or significant disabilities. Therefore, other people within the family (kinship carers), other non-related adults (foster carers/adoptive parents) or the state (social care services) may become the child's key caregivers. For the purposes of this part of the chapter, we will be focusing on 'parents'; however, we recognise that for some children and young people, this may be 'key caregivers'.

To help us understand how influential parents/key caregivers can be, Activity 5.3 focuses on your own personal experiences.

Activity 5.3   Reflection

Building on the reflection exercise in Chapter 4 (Activity 4.1), take a more detailed view of the following elements related to the decisions your parents/key caregivers made for you during your early life stages (pre-conception through to and including childhood and adolescence):

- infant feeding decisions;
- immunisations;
- health screening;
- diet and being active;
- education.

How important do you feel these decisions were in terms of contributing to your health and well-being (both physical and emotional)? Were any decisions made more complex due to social, cultural, religious or personal beliefs and customs? What sources of information (e.g. people, published information, social media) helped them make their decisions? From your personal perspective of these topics, what considerations do you think you might make if you were a parent now?

As this is a personal reflection, no outline answer is given at the end of the chapter.

This activity has hopefully highlighted to you the potential challenges facing parents when making decisions about their children's lives, as well as the influences on these decisions. Parents who have physical, mental and/or cognitive impairments can find making decisions for their children stressful, so compassionate, supportive approaches are essential. For parents whose children have additional or complex needs, these decisions will have added complexity, and the emotional impact on the parents and other family members may be significant.

Decisions are not taken in isolation, with many parents accessing services and published resources in a variety of mediums (e.g. printed, audio, online, mobile apps) to develop their knowledge to make informed decisions, although this requires a level of literacy and ability to understand and process information. Even with good levels of health literacy, the myriad of information available through official and unofficial sources (e.g. social media) can be confusing.

People within the parents' interpersonal and social networks are also influential in decision making. However, their contribution may reflect established family customs and beliefs that are not evidence based. Subsequently, it is necessary for us to have critical awareness of up-to-date evidence and national guidance relating to the health and well-being topic in order to engage in supportive and empowering conversations with families. This aligns with the expectations of the NMC *Code* (2018b). We may also need to respectfully challenge any beliefs that may be founded on misinformation, supporting our conversations with accurate evidence and guiding parents to robust and reliable information.

Infant feeding

A simple choice for parents about what to feed their baby will have an impact on their child's later health and well-being. Infant feeding decisions are considered by parents throughout the antenatal period and have an important role in the health and well-being of their child in terms of both growth and emotional attachment to their parents. Parents, and especially mothers, are not making infant feeding decisions in isolation. The decision can be intensely personal, often linked to the mother's body image and beliefs around being a mother. Family members, including the partner and females within the close personal and social networks, can have a significant impact on the mother's decisions. Furthermore, socio-economic status and social norms, such as public acceptance of breastfeeding, are also influential.

Research summary: The link between infant feeding and obesity

There is an important link between method of infant feeding (breast versus artificial milk) and the rates of obesity in childhood. Evidence suggests that children who have been breastfed may be less likely to be obese as a child and into adulthood than those who have been fed artificial milk. Although the reasons are complex, the potential factors may be related to the differences between breast and artificial milk composition, parent–infant bonding and interaction and feeding regulation differences between infants who are artificially fed or breastfed (Rito et al., 2019).

Supporting families in their infant feeding decisions requires consideration of their personal circumstances and the health of the mother and baby. There is an international commitment to promoting breastfeeding due to the health benefits, with healthcare trusts in the UK achieving 'baby-friendly' status (UNICEF, 2019).

Childhood immunisations

Childhood immunisations are an essential element of public health policies in relation to disease prevention, and parents play an important role in ensuring their children participate in vaccination programmes. Within the UK, there are vaccination schedules for people across the life course, with most vaccinations falling in the childhood years (UK Health Security Agency, 2022).

Childhood infectious diseases can have significant consequences for some individuals, such as life-changing effects or even death. Some childhood infectious diseases, such as measles and rubella, have implications for the wider population because they are highly contagious, and in unvaccinated communities can grow to epidemic proportions. People who are especially vulnerable due to their age and health needs (e.g. newborns, those who are immuno-suppressed) are most at risk of adverse effects or death. Therefore, public health policies aim to reduce or eradicate these diseases to protect vulnerable people within populations. To do this, a substantial number of the population need to be immunised to confer **herd immunity**, thus limiting the transmission of the disease to those who are vulnerable.

However, vaccinations for children and young people are a topic of much debate. Across the UK, there have been cases of measles outbreaks in localised communities and in certain populations such as migrants, travellers, anthroposophic (Steiner) and Orthodox Jewish communities. This is because there was no 'herd immunity' as some children and young people had missed out on vaccinations for a variety of reasons. Some parents have been adversely influenced by the media focus in the late 1990s and early 2000s on the now discredited 'research' by Andrew Wakefield and colleagues linking the measles, mumps and rubella (MMR) vaccination to autism (Godlee et al., 2011). Other reasons include a community's religious or cultural views, the transient lifestyle of a community that has resulted in its members missing out on immunisation clinics, or that an individual's country of origin does not have a robust vaccination schedule and they arrive in the UK unvaccinated (PHE, 2019c).

Subsequently, there are government strategies to increase the uptake of childhood immunisations while maintaining the key messages to the whole population eligible for the various vaccinations. In doing so, the strategy aims to achieve and maintain herd immunity within the population.

Scenario: Engaging in discussions about childhood immunisation choices

While on practice placement, you are sitting in the canteen on your break with two healthcare assistants who are talking about their children. One states that she has received a reminder to get her preschool child immunised. Although her child had the immunisations as a baby, a friend has told her that there is research that says the MMR 'gives children autism'. She is now not sure what to do and asks you what you think.

This is a scenario that is unfortunately not uncommon; therefore, Activity 5.4 will enable you to explore how you might approach this situation.

Activity 5.4   Critical thinking and communication

To critically explore your response to this scenario, consider what do you need to know, and where can you find information on childhood immunisations? What are your personal thoughts/beliefs on childhood immunisations? What are nurses' professional responsibilities in promoting healthy choices? How might you respond?

An outline answer is provided at the end of the chapter.

While you may have found this activity challenging, it is important to be prepared so that you can engage in effective health promotion conversations. People can be presented with a dilemma based on information that has no sound evidential basis but is reflective of wider public perception. Therefore, it is essential that when they seek our guidance, we provide unbiased and consistent messages to support the decision-making process.

Concept summary: NHS health screening

As a preventative health promotion intervention, people are offered health screening across the lifespan. Some screening tests fall in the antenatal and newborn period, so parents will need to make decisions about whether to consent to these for their children.

The premise of health screening is to identify whether people are at higher risk of a health condition and to provide early treatment to stop or limit the progression of the disease. Further tests and interventions are required if the screening test is positive. No health screening is an exact science, with a level of 'false positive' and 'false negative' results occurring. The UK Screening Committee advises Public Health England on recommended screening programmes that are supported by evidence, based on the population reach and effectiveness of the screening.

Diet and being active

The parental choices on the family's diet and exercise impact on not only the physical, but also the psychological development of children and young people. The family approach to diet can be influenced by cultural factors, food traditions passed down through generations or the socio-economic circumstances of the family and their access to basic resources for daily living. As we have briefly considered, infant feeding decisions are important in the very early years in terms of both growth and emotional development. Once the child is weaned, developing healthy eating habits through childhood continues to be influenced by parental choices. Family eating habits that favour high-fat, high-sugar food and drink, as well as a lack of exercise, can adversely impact on weight. This raises the potential of the child (and other family members) becoming overweight or obese, and in turn impacts on the child's immediate and long-term health and self-image (Office for Health Improvement & Disparities, 2022a).

As we have seen in Chapter 4, poor diet and exercise increases the risk of developing health conditions that can have a significant negative impact on well-being and life expectancy, so it is important to reinforce positive health behaviours with families. National public health campaigns such as Better Health provide resources that promote the important role of parents in the diet and exercise decisions impacting on their children (Better Health, 2021). We will explore the policies driving public health campaigns in Chapter 7.

Education

An essential element in a person's social and emotional development is their access to education. A parent's personal education levels, as well as their views on education for their children, have a significant impact on their child's development. In areas of socio-economic deprivation, the rates of children and young people not in education or subsequent training increase. The important Marmot Review (Marmot, 2010) identified that children and young people who have had poor engagement with education during their childhood were more likely to experience negative impacts on health and personal literacy, with limited employment potential and subsequently lower economic stability. Just ten years later, the COVID-19 pandemic has brought the significance of access to education into stark focus. Marmot et al. (2020) asserts that children and young people from deprived families have been disproportionately affected in terms of poorer access to education and learning materials during the national lockdowns, with the concern that this will lead to worse outcomes for people from deprived communities.

Parental behaviours

Parental behaviours have an impact on their child's health and well-being. Social and emotional well-being is developed from the very early stages throughout childhood. Parents have a key role in this process, through the early bonding and attachment, as well as nurturing the child's self-esteem and self-image.

Parents act as key role models, modelling behaviours relating to a range of emotional, physical, mental and social elements. However, parents' own emotional, psychological and physical health will have an impact on the child. Parents with mental ill health may not be emotionally available to develop strong attachment bonds with their children, and this may have a lasting impact on the child's emotional development. Similarly, parents who have significant physical or mental health needs may have to rely on their partner and children to support their own health needs, which impacts on the family dynamics and the developmental needs of the child. If they are solo parenting then this will have a direct impact on their children. Children who have a caring role may need to take on responsibilities beyond their age (e.g. intimate care of the parent) or be unable to regularly attend school, which impacts on their educational attainment (Chikhradze, Knecht & Metzing, 2017).

Parental health behaviours can also have an impact on their children. Parents who engage in physical activity and healthy eating choices will have a positive influence on their children. Conversely, parents who engage in unhealthy behaviours can influence their child's behaviour in adolescence and early adulthood. An example of this is parental cigarette smoking, with evidence suggesting that smoking is socially reinforced. Adolescents of smoking parents are 80 per cent more likely to commence smoking than those who live in non-smoking households (ONS, 2017).

Adulthood

Working age and adult life stage (16–64 years old)

Family dynamics change during adulthood, with people forming social bonds with new partners, increasing their support networks and potentially expanding their own families by having children. Adult family members who have mental capacity are also able to make their own decisions in relation to lifestyle choices, vaccinations, health screening and health and well-being-related activities. Some adults will have lifelong health conditions diagnosed in childhood or from birth and will continue to need support from their family network and the wider adult health and social care provision. However, as in the opening case study, if these adults have capacity, they will now lead the decision making relating to their physical, social and emotional needs.

During this life stage, many health conditions can impact on individuals that have a correlation to early life decisions. As we have seen, early feeding decisions, immunisation choices, diet, exercise, educational opportunities and parental health behaviours will impact on individuals throughout their lives. In particular, poorer diet and exercise decisions can raise a person's risk of developing health conditions that may have long-term impacts, such as type 2 diabetes or heart disease. Ethnicity may also be a factor, with some ethnic groups being more at risk of type 2 diabetes and associated health conditions at lower body mass index (BMI) levels (PHE, 2018a). Many of these conditions are diagnosed during adulthood, particularly if they continue the lifestyle patterns of their childhood and may impact them for the rest of their lives. Some of these conditions will result in shorter lifespan or poorer quality of life for the individual (Steel et al., 2018), and will subsequently impact on their family.

Risk taking

Some health needs emerge during this life stage that are unrelated to childhood elements, including new risk-taking behaviours. Young adults in particular may also make life decisions that do not reflect their parents' decisions during their childhood. Once away from the influence of their parents, young adults may develop risk-taking behaviours and make decisions regarding alcohol, unprotected sex (increasing the risk of sexually transmitted infections and unplanned pregnancy), smoking and illicit drug use, which can impact on their physical and mental health and well-being. As we have seen, whatever the stage of adulthood, some of these health behaviours can influence family members, especially children, as well as the life expectancy of the adult.

Employment and health

While health needs can impact on people's employment, for some people their occupation may carry risks to their health, such as being in the armed forces, heavy industry or sedentary jobs. Evidence suggests that health conditions can affect the employment status of the family member and have an adverse impact on their economic stability and ability to provide for themselves and their family. Individuals who are able to work but have health needs may be less productive when in work or have more days off work due to illness. This impacts on not only their family's financial stability, but potentially the productivity and economic stability of the company they work for, and in turn the wider economy.

Older people (adults over 64 years old)

From a health promotion perspective, there is an importance in focusing on the wellness of people in their later years of life, taking an asset-based approach. Consideration of the resources available to the older person in personal, social, economic and environmental areas of their life enables identification of health and well-being needs and resources (Hornby-Turner et al., 2017). Personal factors will relate to physical and mental health needs and the person's perceptions of their health status. Social factors relate to the social network, the availability of resources and the willingness and ability of the person to engage with the network. Economic factors may have an influence on the physical and social well-being of the person. Evidence shows that people in this life stage who are financially stable age more successfully, being able to access a variety of social activities and maintain a good standard of living. Finally, environmental factors relate to people's local geographical area and the natural environment. How people can access, interact with and enjoy their local area will impact their physical and emotional health and well-being.

Carers

A key consideration in this life stage is the increasing impact on family members if they become carers to relatives with progressive and life-limiting conditions. Nevertheless, it is important to recognise that both children and adults can become carers. The Department for Work and Pensions *Family Resources Survey* (DWP, 2020) identified that the majority of carers (34 per cent) were adult children caring for their parents, with 18 per cent caring for their partners. However, these statistics may not present the true picture, as some people may not identify as a 'carer', seeing their caring role as integral to the family or cultural traditions.

Being a carer for a family member has far-reaching implications. Adult children may be caring for one or both of their parents in addition to a full-time job or studentship or be unable to work or undertake further study due to significant care needs of their parents or other adult relatives. Older people caring for their partners may have health and well-being needs of their own, or neglect their own health needs to look after their partner. Therefore, we need to be mindful of the health and well-being of the carer themselves when providing care to the family member with health needs (SCIE, 2019).

Analysis by the Scottish Government (2015) has identified that carers may experience fatigue, musculoskeletal problems and exhaustion as they often provide 24-hour care. This may contribute to deteriorating mental health, with the caring role being linked to increased levels of carer stress, anxiety and depression. There may also be deteriorations in the carer's physical health as a result of neglecting their own health needs, including missing or delaying appointments or health screening.

Although there are statutory requirements to support carers embedded within the Care Act 2014, a review of social care by the King's Fund identified that direct support from local councils had declined while applications for Carer's Allowance had risen (Bottery et al., 2019). This highlights the increasing challenge of access to resources for informal, unpaid carers within family units.

Family coping and resilience

As we have seen, families have a significant influence and impact on their members' health and well-being throughout the life course. Most people cope well with the changing patterns and challenges of daily life, as well as the changing stages of human development, subsequently adapting to socially accepted role expectations. However, health needs that require people to reframe and then navigate the challenges of a socially or culturally accepted view of life, health and death will create stressors, which challenges a family's coping mechanisms.

Families where individual members may have specific needs and require relatives to become informal carers (e.g. long-term conditions, learning disabilities, physical disabilities, mental health needs) will impact on family members' personal, emotional and social resources, particularly when the relative may have multiple needs (Lee and Roberts, 2018). Therefore, supporting families to develop coping strategies is integral to the nursing role.

There are many theories that help us to consider human coping and resilience when confronted with stressful situations. Perhaps the most well-known is Lazarus and Folkman's (1984) theory of stress and coping, which considers problem-focused versus emotion-based coping mechanisms. Problem-focused approaches are more likely to result in adaptive behaviours because individuals actively attempt to assess and understand what the stressor is, as well as their internal and external resources that will help them to cope. Individuals whose coping mechanisms are driven by emotions believe they cannot address the source of the stress, resulting in increased psychological stress. The aim of family-centred approaches is to promote coping strategies and resilience to enable the family to be empowered to regain balance, focusing on strengths to develop positive adaptive approaches to cope with actual and potential changes to health and well-being (Lee and Roberts, 2018).

To support your developing awareness of this aspect of family health promotion, Activity 5.5 will explore family coping from your practice experiences.

Activity 5.5   Critical thinking

Consider a family from your practice experience who were coping with a family member with a long-term health need.

Taking a social ecological perspective, what are the factors that could influence their coping and resilience?

An outline answer is available at the end of the chapter.

Hopefully, this activity enabled you to identify potential strengths as well as perhaps considering some of the challenges facing families, particularly when there are deteriorations in people's health and well-being. Engaging with families is essential to wider behaviour change and sustained management of people's health and well-being. Developing awareness of family strengths and needs is important to this process, although there may be challenges nurses will need to manage in order to support families effectively. Family dynamics, social, religious and cultural influences, poverty and deprivation and entrenched beliefs about their health behaviours are significantly influential to people's health needs and can present barriers that nurses and other health professionals will need to manage sensitively. Some family members may have their own physical and emotional health and well-being needs that impact on their personal resources to cope with their relative's needs. Understanding the elements that impact on coping and resilience within families requires us to consider and appreciate the perspective of each key family member.

Similar to the healthcare approaches we explored in Chapter 4, being person-centred, empowering and developing actions and finding solutions that are developed *with* the person and their family are important to successful coping strategies. This includes collaborative goal setting and utilising statutory and community resources to support the family. Of course, moving people's thinking towards positive problem-solving behaviours can take time, and people's physical and mental well-being can significantly influence the development of positive adaptive behaviours.

Recognition of the resources within families to increase their resilience and enable them to cope with their health and well-being needs is an essential element in effective provision of care. People with long-term health needs may experience years of fluctuating health, including the deterioration of their health and well-being over time. The ability to be resilient and adapt to these fluctuations will define whether families can function and cope effectively.

Chapter summary

This chapter focused on the importance of families within health promotion. We clarified what health education is and considered the importance of health literacy to effective health education activities. In taking a life course perspective, we explored the influence of families on the health and well-being of their family members. Finally, we considered factors that influence effective coping and resilience within families.

Activities: Brief outline answers

Activity 5.1   Reflection (page 68)

There are many topics, but you may have considered education relating to a long-term condition, self-care post operation, medication administration, sexual health education, and toileting.

Individual and family elements may also be challenges:

- age and level of literacy;
- willingness to participate (e.g. consider behaviour change models/self-efficacy);
- communication needs (e.g. related to health, life stage, language);
- venue, time and resources;
- family dynamics;
- socio-economic factors (e.g. finances, transport, resources at home – perhaps requiring occupational therapy involvement).

Activity 5.2   Critical thinking and communication (page 70)

Rosie has a mild learning difficulty, and her cerebral palsy limits her gross and fine motor movements in her arms and hands. However, we should never assume that people with physical and/or learning disabilities are not capable of learning new skills, even if they may need to adapt the skill to take their needs into consideration. To enhance this intervention, you may like to suggest that Rosie's partner could also participate in an education session to promote shared responsibility.

To conduct an effective health education intervention, combining 'teach back' and 'chunk and check' would be beneficial – remember, Rosie will set the pace of the interaction. Your communication approach should include:

- *Check*: Establishing what Rosie knows already. This allows you to assess knowledge and is important in providing person-centred care.
- *Chunk & check 2/teach back*: Showing her the condom packet and how to check the expiry date. Showing her how to open the condom packet and how to hold the condom. Support Rosie to practise this herself, checking her knowledge as she practises. This requires a level of dexterity and Rosie may need a few attempts to work out a way to do this. If Rosie feels this would be too difficult, you can suggest that her partner could take this role as part of foreplay.
- *Chunk 3/teach back*: Talking to her about things that may degrade or pierce the condom (e.g. jewellery, oils).
- *Chunk 4/teach back/check*: Demonstrating putting on and safe disposal of a condom using the condom demonstrator. This may take time and several attempts to allow Rosie to work out how to accommodate any fine motor function deficits.

Activity 5.4   Critical thinking and communication (page 74)

Resources: There are various governmental resources relating to immunisations and immunisation schedules. A key resource is the *Green Book* (UK Government, 2021).

Communication: Finding out from the person what exactly they are concerned about and what information they have accessed is an important first step. Empowering people to make decisions will require you to have a sound knowledge of the information and the options available. Signposting people to information and key professionals (e.g. health visitor, practice nurse, GP) will also assist them in making their decisions.

Professionalism: You may have your own personal views on various health topics such as childhood vaccinations, which may challenge your belief systems and provide you with a personal dilemma. Nurses are bound to uphold the values of *The Code*, and therefore we must always provide care that reflects the best available evidence, setting clear boundaries between our personal beliefs and professional requirements (NMC, 2018b). As parents will often turn to health professionals for information and advice on immunisations, contributing to an unbiased and informed discussion is vital (UK Health Security Agency, 2019).

Activity 5.5   Critical thinking (page 79)

There are many potential factors influencing coping and resilience. Hopefully, you have considered:

- the physical and mental health of family members including multi-morbidities and deteriorating long-term conditions;
- family dynamics (e.g. cohesive, strong/weak bonds, communication channels, location to each other);
- available family resources (e.g. personal skills and abilities – including health literacy – emotional resilience, beliefs and values, material resources such as housing and finances);
- the potential wider influences on the family, such as cultural/religious beliefs and values and social expectations (e.g. is the health need taboo among the religious/cultural group? Are there cultural/social expectations on caring and coping?);
- political and policy factors (e.g. provision and access to services and welfare policies such as benefits).

Useful websites

www.gov.uk/topic/population-screening-programmes

For further information on health screening in the UK and information on population screening programmes, you can visit the UK government website or Public Health England's blog.

www.instituteofhealthequity.org/resources-reports/build-back-fairer-the-covid-19-marmot-review

Build Back Fairer: The COVID-19 Marmot Review: The Pandemic, Socioeconomic and Health Inequalities in England (Marmot et al 2022) This is an important report that provides insight into the impact of the pandemic on the population in England.

Chapter 6   Health promotion at a community level

(Continued)

Platform 7: Co-ordinating care

At the point of registration, the registered nurse will be able to:

7.1　understand and apply the principles of partnership, collaboration and inter-agency working across all relevant sectors.

7.2　understand health legislation and current health and social care policies, and the mechanisms involved in influencing policy development and change, differentiating where appropriate between the devolved legislatures of the United Kingdom.

Chapter aims

After reading this chapter, you will be able to:

- define community and how people engage within it;
- identify why communities are important to the health and well-being of its members, including those from **marginalised** populations;
- consider ways to effectively engage with communities;
- consider how community engagement can impact on healthcare provision.

Introduction

In the previous two chapters, we have taken a social ecological perspective to explore health promotion, first focusing on individuals and then on families. In this chapter, we will focus on health promotion at the community level.

Case study: George and Oluchi

George and Oluchi retired two years ago after living and working in London for most of their adult lives. They have moved to the Midlands and are getting used to living in a new community.

George and I decided to move to be with George's extended family in Birmingham when our children left home and moved away from London. Being from Nigeria, we wanted to be with the Nigerian community here as our culture and our community is very important to us. Our church has supported us to feel settled, and we have made new friends and reconnected with old ones. The added benefit of living with a community that reflects our cultural roots is that there are shops such as food and clothing markets that sell Nigerian products. There is also a shared sense of culture among the local people and social activities reflect this. This connects us to our homeland while at the same time we support each other to live successfully in the UK.

This case study highlights the potential benefits of belonging to a community. We all develop relationships with people and groups with whom we have affiliations, either because of family links or within social, cultural and/or religious networks. These groups may have particular health and well-being needs, perhaps linked to their location (e.g. access to green spaces such as local parks, air pollution in inner-city areas), socially accepted health behaviours (e.g. regional or ethnic food culture, or social activities with social norms around drinking alcohol, illicit drug use and/or smoking), wider determinants of health (e.g. deprivation, **poverty**) or a health need relating to ethnicity (e.g. body mass differences between ethnic groups increasing obesity risks).

In this chapter, we will explore what we mean by communities and why they are important in contributing to the health and well-being of their members. We will consider how communities may shape the future of health within healthcare, through empowering community groups to lead on addressing the health and well-being needs of their members. Within this element, we will explore the perspectives of communities who are marginalised, identifying specific areas in which key health needs have been identified and the importance of supporting these communities to have a voice. Finally, a theme running throughout the chapter will be the importance of working with communities to meet the changing needs of health service provision.

What is a community?

NICE (2017:6) states *A community is a group of people who have common characteristics or interests. Communities can be defined by: geographical location, race, ethnicity, age, occupation, a shared interest or affinity (such as religion and faith) or other common bonds, such as health need or disadvantage. People who are socially isolated are also considered to be a community group.*

Using this definition, it is important to consider the range of communities that exist in the geographical areas that we live and work in, as well as their potential needs.

Activity 6.1   Critical thinking

Based on the definition above, how many different communities in the area where you live can you identify? Are they place-based or groups with members who have a common identity? Where would you look to find information? Choose one community to explore further. Consider their needs when accessing healthcare. What knowledge would help you to provide optimum care to people from this community?

An outline answer is provided at the end of the chapter.

This activity has hopefully highlighted the wealth of groups and communities that exist in your areas of practice. The word 'community' engenders a sense of belonging-ness and a common focus with the people who are members of the community. We all belong to various communities, whether it is the village or street we live in or a group with whom we have social, religious or cultural affiliations. In fact, as student nurses, you are part of a group, both within your own university and within the wider student nurse community in the UK.

Activity 6.2 will enable you to explore the benefits of being a member of the student nurse community, as well as the potential impacts on your health and well-being.

Activity 6.2 Reflection

Reflect on your membership of the student nurse community in the UK.

What do you get from being a part of the student nurse community? Do you engage with your community on a university, local or national level (or all of these levels)? If so, what activities do you get involved in, and why? If not, why not? Does being part of the student nurse community impact on your health and well-being? If so, in what ways? If not, why not?

An outline answer is provided at the end of the chapter.

Hopefully, focusing on your membership of the student nurse community has enabled you to consider how important it is to be part of such a group. As you will have seen from your engagement in Activity 6.1, there are multiple groups and communities. People have a variety of reasons why they become members of groups or live in certain communities, including support, advice and a common goal. Some communities have a specific function and role for their members, and there are others that perform an additional function within wider society such as charitable groups.

It is important to understand how communities may impact on the health and well-being of their members so that we can target health promotion effectively, and (perhaps more importantly) engage and empower the community in setting their own priorities to address their health needs proactively. In fact, this topic has grown in importance over recent years, partly influenced by the need to reframe health services to meet the needs of the diverse UK population, but also in response to the ongoing financial review of health service provision. While the COVID-19 pandemic placed financial and resourcing pressures on health and social care services, it also provided an insight into how communities worked together to support their members. Subsequently, there has been increasing interest in exploring how community engagement and empowerment can support statutory service delivery in ways that are innovative, cost-effective, sustainable and fit for purpose.

How do communities impact on the health and well-being of their members?

As we have seen in Chapter 4, from a social ecological perspective, people are impacted by multiple elements within their lives, including personal, social, cultural and political influences. Communities have the potential to influence individuals both positively and negatively. Positive elements include shared skills, shared resources and assets, shared knowledge, shared beliefs and values and shared responsibilities.

Membership of a community can have positive effects in terms of increasing knowledge and literacy, as well as in identifying, developing and using resources (both material and emotional resources) for the benefit of its members and the wider population in which the community functions. Communities can also be responsible for change, whether in terms of individual behaviours (e.g. smoking cessation, or increased engagement with vaccination and screening programmes) or to benefit the community as a whole, including community empowerment and having a stronger collective voice to raise the profile of community issues.

Public Health England highlights the wider contribution of community development and participation to citizenship, including increasing democracy and community empowerment to mobilise resources and assets. This ultimately results in the development of services that are effective and sustainable (PHE, 2018b).

Nevertheless, for some people, living in a community can be challenging. Communities may have expectations on the commitment and engagement of their members that potentially disadvantage or isolate people whose resources are limited (whether personal, financial or material). In many geographical communities, there is a social gradient that may exclude certain individuals or groups from the provision of activities and resources due to factors such as limited literacy, limited financial resources, poverty, unemployment or disabilities. Therefore, the wider determinants of health are an important consideration when exploring the impact of health and well-being on the members of any community.

Box 6.1 Report overview

The Marmot Review (Marmot, 2010) presented a stark picture of people's experience of living in the UK. The review highlighted the impact of the social gradient of health on the population, particularly the impact for people and communities who experience social deprivation. It has long been acknowledged that there are sectors of the population who are marginalised and where health and social inequalities result in poorer health and well-being outcomes for people. Members of communities living in social deprivation experience poverty and have poorer access to and engagement with education, employment, services and local resources. This can negatively affect their aspirations and social mobility, and

(Continued)

(Continued)

these combined elements impact on health, well-being and life expectancy. Lord Marmot and his team proposed six policy objectives to reduce inequalities and improve the health and well-being of the population:

1. Give every child the best start in life.
2. Enable all children, young people and adults to maximise their capabilities and have control over their lives.
3. Create fair employment and good work for all.
4. Ensure a healthy standard of living for all.
5. Create and develop healthy and sustainable places and communities.
6. Strengthen the role and impact of ill health prevention.

You will notice that one of the key objectives was to create and develop healthy and sustainable places and communities. Essential to this objective is the national and local approach to the following elements:

- *Policies that reduce health inequalities and reduce climate change*: This element included addressing transport policies, taking environmental action, protecting and providing green spaces, policies to improve the 'food environment' in local areas (e.g. availability of nutritious food at affordable prices), reducing fuel poverty and policies that promote the building of energy-efficient homes.
- *Developing integrated policies that focus on planning, transport, housing, environmental and health policies to address the social determinants of health*: This element focused on the strategic approaches to the provision of key elements within community developments. The report cited that integration of these policies could reduce inequalities and improve the health and well-being of local populations.
- *Improving community capital*: This element focused on the way that communities define and shape themselves, as well as how local and national policies and structures recognise and support this development. This is important because in deprived areas, engagement in community life is limited, with less volunteering due to lack of resources, high crime and poor levels of community cohesion. People can become isolated, experiencing high levels of stress, deprivation and poverty, and have limited social networks to support them. The Marmot Review recognised that community capital was essential to empowering communities, reducing isolation through activities that developed **social capital**, in turn strengthening bonds, increasing trust and reciprocity. Therefore, a key focus would be to develop policies to support sustainable community development and reduce inequalities.

Since its publication, the health inequalities which Marmot (2010) reported have been intensified by the impact of the COVID-19 pandemic on every aspect of public life. More people in our communities are experiencing poverty, including those with a regular income who have a gap between their wages and the cost of living. This demonstrates the ongoing need to be aware of how inequalities impact on us and the people in our communities, and how collective action is needed (Marmot et al., 2020).

Following the Marmot Review in 2010, legislation was passed which placed a legal duty on health services and local authorities to reduce inequalities and consider the communities in which the key agencies provide services:

- The Health and Social Care Act 2012 placed a legal duty on health bodies and services to reduce health inequalities; this included public health service provision moving to local authorities.
- The Public Services (Social Value) Act 2012 placed a legal duty on local authorities to commission services and policies that were mindful of economic, environmental and social well-being.

To help us understand the way that local councils enact these legal duties, we can explore local government websites for information on local strategies and initiatives. To assist you in developing this awareness, Activity 6.3 requires you to focus on a UK local authority area that you are familiar with.

Activity 6.3 Critical thinking

For this activity, we would like you to focus on a location within the UK with which you are very familiar, such as the county where your family home or university is situated.

Access and explore the county or local council website for this area. Can you identify the ways in which community engagement occurs? How have the council approached supporting and empowering communities? What health and well-being targets have they set? Can you see how the legal Acts that we have highlighted previously have aimed to influence local policies to reduce inequalities in health and deprivation (consider social, environmental and economic well-being)?

An outline answer is provided at the end of the chapter.

Hopefully, this activity has enabled you to have an awareness of the diverse needs of local communities, as well as the policies and services that are influencing them. This is essential in how we approach the provision of care for both people and the communities within which they live. Local and national policies will shape how the services we work within are provided, as well as where resources are focused. However, increasingly, many of these services are being influenced and co-created by the communities themselves.

Community empowerment

As you will have noticed from the previous chapters, taking an empowering person- and family-centred approach is central to successful health interventions. Working with communities is a further extension of this approach, aiming to strengthen community assets for the health and well-being of community membership. Community empowerment embraces the collective participation of community members to not only shape services, but also engage in developing and participating in sustainable developments.

Salutogenesis

Salutogenesis is a theoretical approach to understanding the complexity of community empowerment, encompassing an asset-based approach, primarily focusing on the fundamental resources and capacities of people and the causes of health rather than the causes of disease. It concentrates on an 'upstream' approach whereby people within communities are empowered to identify their own needs and are supported to address them. This creates community-driven sustainable solutions which are much more effective than services deciding what is best for the communities that they serve (Lindstrom, 2020). A particular benefit of salutogenesis is attributed to the mental well-being of individuals within the community. This includes strengthening self-efficacy and resilience at an individual level, which, when replicated, results in community-wide connectedness, resilience and empowerment.

This is particularly important in communities where there may be a culture of learned helplessness, low motivation, isolation and poor health outcomes, such as those with high levels of deprivation. Communities that are marginalised are at a particular disadvantage as, individually, people may have low self-efficacy and limited personal and material resources, which creates a sense of powerlessness.

The impact of living in a marginalised community

People who live in communities that are on the periphery of the mainstream social group can experience disadvantages, and therefore are marginalised within the society in which they live. Traditionally, we may think of marginalised communities as those that include people who have specific cultural, sexual or religious characteristics, such as people included within the protected characteristics as defined by the Equality Act 2010. Nevertheless, it is important to appreciate that marginalisation is not one element and can include a combination of elements that contribute to a group being marginalised. Imagine if you were living in poverty and had none of the basic resources available to the majority of the population, such as access to affordable accommodation, food, fuel, money, transportation and social support groups. You may also derive from a lower socio-economic group, and subsequently may be viewed as having a lower social value than the rest of the wider community, leaving you feeling isolated. Furthermore, you may also be stigmatised because you are from a group that does not 'conform' to the accepted societal norms (e.g. sexual orientation at odds with your community's religious views) or you are disabled, and therefore experience stigma and restrictions on access to employment, services and resources. You may not be able to speak the language of the mainstream population and find it difficult to navigate services and resources. You may be homeless or live in temporary accommodation.

You may also be unemployed or unable to find work, which limits your available house-hold finances and potentially places you and those you live with at risk of living in poverty.

It is not unusual for areas within the UK to have several marginalised communities in one locality, and therefore there is competing demand for resources and services. People living in some communities may find it difficult to have a voice and their own social networks may be limited. They may not trust the local authorities because services may be complicated to navigate and the established systems (e.g. housing, benefits) may be perceived as discriminatory, presenting a barrier. Those communities that are empowered and can articulate their needs are in a stronger position to secure resources and funding to develop services. Therefore, this presents a challenge for all service providers, whether statutory or voluntary, in meeting the needs of the populations they serve in a fair and equitable way.

The impact of deprivation

It is known that people from disadvantaged communities have poorer health and well-being outcomes. Foster et al. (2018) conducted a large UK population-based cohort study, which identified that there was a higher risk of poorer health outcomes for people who experience socio-economic deprivation. The study explored the link between health behaviours (smoking, alcohol use, diet, physical activity, combined with emerging risk factors of sleep duration and television watching time), health outcomes and socio-economic status. It concluded that people living in low socio-economic groups were at a disproportionately higher risk of the effects of health behaviour risk factors than people from other socio-economic groups. The report suggested that a combination of factors may be contributing to increased morbidity and mortality risk for people living in socio-economic deprivation. The combination of health behaviours, the psychological stress of living in deprivation and reduced access to health services potentially increase the vulnerability of people living in deprived groups.

Studies such as this underline the importance of working with communities in an empowering way to develop individual and group resilience, as well as providing sustainable services. However, traditionally, service provision may be responsive to a particular need rather than proactively supporting long-term community health and well-being. Marginalised communities may receive targeted interventions to address a specific need following peaks of a particular health and well-being issue that has impacted members of their communities. This could be a measles outbreak, such as those we discussed in Chapter 5, a cluster of deaths related to illicit drug use, a high rate of teenage pregnancy in a particular locality or increasing rates of knife crime and related injuries and deaths within youth groups in inner-city areas. However, this approach is problematic in that it responds to a deficit rather than being forward focused to address the underpinning elements of the problem in a long-term, preventative way.

An asset or deficit approach to healthcare provision?

The ultimate aim of community empowerment is that the membership is empowered to identify and contribute to resolving key issues and needs impacting their community. Communities need to have a voice, and therefore it is important that there is a committed, rather than tokenistic, approach to engagement from local authorities and service providers. Power and dynamics within established national and local systems and policies need to change to embrace this approach.

Deficit-based approach to health provision

The well-established systems of national and local government policy, funding and service provision traditionally reflect a top-down hierarchical approach to policymaking and service delivery. Services are provided to meet an overall need, driven by data that highlight where deficits exist. Government policies aim to provide adequate funding where it is needed most, raising taxes and setting guiding principles for local authorities and integrated health and social care systems (UK Government 2022).

A deficit-based approach to service provision in healthcare can be problematic for a number of reasons. First, the professional perspective of the problem and the solution may differ significantly from that of the members of the community. Second, the focus of the intervention may not be the focus of what the community values as important and the key need at the time. Finally, the proposed solution may be time-limited and funding/ resources may limit the effectiveness and reach to members of the targeted community.

Subsequently, sustained improvements are not realised, and services may be poorly used. Within healthcare, this can result in services that respond to emerging pockets of local need in a reactionary way, creating services or resources that are often time-limited due to short-term funding and do not meet the long-term needs of the population they intend to serve.

Financial constraints on health service providers may result in the imposing of limitations to services, changes in the way services are provided and accessed, and review of staffing skill ratios, which potentially impact on the quality of the service delivery.

Case study: A deficit approach to health service delivery

Jude is a senior nurse who works in a community mental healthcare team. He is acutely aware that nationally, the demand for Mental Health Services has been gradually increasing over several years. In his local community, since the start of the COVID-19 pandemic, the demand has now exceeded the capacity of the health services currently available. Historically, the national austerity measures have seen statutory mental health service provision streamlined into smaller teams of staff who cover large localities. Jude tells us about a recent initiative to support service provision to people in mental health crisis:

Recently, we have seen an escalation in the number of people experiencing exacerbations of their mental health condition and a rise in new referrals. We couldn't keep up with the service demands and the local A&E services were seeing increasing numbers of people in mental health crisis. The staffing levels in the Trust were unable to cope with the influx of people needing acute interventions as well as those people already receiving community Mental Health Services in their own homes. We raised this with senior managers, but we had been told that as yet, no additional funding, staff or resources are available.

The Trust managers decided that in order for the Mental Health Services to meet the increasing demands, the community provision should be temporarily reconfigured. People who were receiving ongoing follow-up visits in their homes were asked to visit a clinic or have online consultations. This released staff who were travelling between patients' homes for one-to-one visits. The managers believed this would create a more manageable centralised service provision and would help those patients receiving ongoing care to demonstrate their engagement with their treatment. Part of the community mental health team were diverted to provide short-term support to people in crisis to try to reduce the numbers of people attending A&E.

We have just reviewed this change after eight weeks. This has revealed that the number of people who are long-term patients recorded higher rates of non-attendance at the follow-up clinics or no-shows on the online consultations. The rates of people attending A&E in crisis has escalated, with many of the people visiting A&E being patients with long-term mental health conditions. Some patients have said they missed the face-to-face interactions with nurses.

This case study presents a deficit approach to managing health service provision. The result of the change to service provision, while aiming to increase the effectiveness of the resource at a time of increasing need, ultimately results in isolating sectors of the community that require services. However, taking an asset-based approach may begin to develop long-term sustainable community resources, supporting local statutory service provision.

Asset-based approach

Asset-based approaches promote the social capital within the community to meet the needs of the population. The Marmot Review (Marmot, 2010) asserts that social capital is important to sustained change within communities. Importantly, strong social capital has been attributed to individual and community well-being, as well as building community resilience (UKHSA, 2022b).

Asset-based approaches focus on building community assets, not only identifying needs, but also engaging individuals within communities to collectively and actively address community issues. Asset-based approaches raise the health and well-being of the community in numerous ways. Planned initiatives addressing a specific health need in disadvantaged groups are effective in addressing health behaviours, improving self-efficacy and health and well-being outcomes. Individual engagement in their community, such as volunteering, raises individual and collective well-being and strengthens citizenship. Finally, increasing family and social support networks reduces social isolation, improves resilience and has improved health outcomes for individuals (PHE, 2018b).

Working with communities requires a change in the approach of statutory services in terms of both the way they engage with people as well as the design and delivery of services. You may already be familiar with public engagement activities within your local authority area, where local people will contribute to discussions about service delivery.

Figure 6.1 Visual overview of approaches to supporting communities to improve their health (Buck and Wenzel, 2018)

Reproduced with permission from the King's Fund

This may be as simple as canvassing people in a survey, to engaging groups of people in focus group discussions about services provided to the local population. While this approach contributes to service design and provision, there may still be a disproportionate balance of 'power' between the service provider and the community in terms of the final decisions about resource provision.

Asset-based approaches are aimed at engaging and empowering communities to take a more active role in the development of services to meet the needs of the population. Statutory services define the boundaries in which service provision may be designed, but communities are involved in the development, commissioning and delivery of services. Figure 6.1 shows that changing the provision and design of services from service-led to community-led will empower communities to identify and commission services that meet the needs of the community.

It is also suggested that effectively using individual and community assets to improve health and well-being on a wide scale can be cost-effective.

Case study: Services and communities working together – an asset-based approach

The Wigan Deal

In 2011, Wigan Council had a significant funding deficit as a result of national government funding cuts, which resulted in an innovative approach to addressing the needs of the local population while maintaining local services. To address this funding need, Wigan Council took an asset-based approach across all council departments to address the challenges they faced.

The main premise of the 'Deal' is the commitment of all statutory and voluntary services, local businesses and the population in addressing the needs of the area (Wigan Council, 2019). Their staff were given the support to work closely with local community groups to innovate new ways to address needs. It included people being empowered to take responsibility for their own health and well-being and for the way they use local services, as well as funding being provided to groups to meet a community-defined need. The 'Deal' has been successful because people from communities and the key agencies have been empowered to shape the way in which policies are created and services are provided. Local groups have been funded to provide innovative resources based on community-identified needs. This includes:

- Incredible Edible, which received funding to undertake various activities throughout the council area to engage people of all ages in growing their own fruit and vegetables. An intergenerational element of the project aims to reduce loneliness and isolation and improve health and well-being.

(Continued)

(Continued)

- The Blair Project, a social enterprise project supporting young people to develop skills and confidence in science, engineering and digital technology through motorsport activities.
- Adult mentor volunteering, encouraging adults to volunteer to support at-risk young people to reach their potential.
- Training people to become a health champion to promote health and well-being with people within their family or workplace, or a mental health champion to reduce stigma and signpost people in need.

It is important to note that this approach is not a simple and quick solution to the funding issues the council faced. It has been recognised that the commitment of all key partners and the community itself have been essential in driving forward change (Naylor and Wellings, 2019).

This case study is just one example of how local areas can engage with communities successfully to develop and provide services. You may have found more community projects when you undertook Activity 6.3. Local authorities have been encouraged to embrace an asset-based approach, so there may be many activities within their catchment area that increase community engagement and have the health and well-being of the population as a key health target. The UKHSA (2022b) have collated other examples of asset-based approaches from other locations within the UK which you may find interesting (see the end of this chapter for the link).

How can we support community asset-based approaches?

The Wigan Deal highlights the importance of multi-agency working to support the asset-based approach. As nurses, we can engage in community asset-based approaches by working closely with our multi-agency colleagues and the communities in which we work and live. Healthcare practitioners may use community assets and voluntary organisations to refer people to non-clinical services with an aim to improve their health and well-being. This is commonly termed 'social prescribing' (Calderón-Larrañaga et al., 2022). Therefore, knowing what services and activities are already in place is important to support the people we care for on a daily basis. In your nursing role you may be instrumental in supporting individuals in the community to identify their needs and advocate for change.

Activity 6.4 requires you to take an asset-based approach to service provision within communities to which you provide health services.

Activity 6.4   Leadership and management

Focus on a specific group of people to whom your field of nursing provides services; this may be a place-based group or a group with a particular affiliation (e.g. people with a specific health condition, disability, communication needs, or age-related service need).

Taking an asset-based perspective, what community services are available to this population? What range of services and activities can be accessed to improve their health and well-being? What sources can you use to find these services and activities? How can you utilise this knowledge to improve care provision when you are in clinical practice? Reflect on how easy or difficult it was for you to find this information. Consider how the accessibility of resources would impact on people from marginalized groups. What do you think needs to happen to make resources more accessible?

An outline answer is provided at the end of the chapter.

As you may have identified in this activity, there are a range of community services available that can enhance your service provision. Signposting is perhaps one of the most important activities we can do as nurses to empower people across the lifespan to access services and activities that meet their needs. Therefore, having an awareness of the local community needs, assets and resources can assist us in working with communities in a multi-agency and community-focused way to provide services and resources.

There are numerous ways that people's health and well-being can be improved that will also have an impact on a community level. As we have seen in Chapters 4 and 5, empowering people is important in improving health and well-being. While statutory service provision is often the first step in improving health and well-being, people can be engaged in providing services within their communities that support others with their health and well-being needs. These activities strengthen citizenship and develop community capital, building individual and group resilience within communities.

People as assets

Many people within communities act as volunteers, peer supporters or health educators (UKHSA, 2022b). Others may have useful assets (e.g. knowledge, experience, time, social connections) but have not yet engaged in community-based activities. Understanding local opportunities can assist health professionals in not only actively engaging with people to develop services, but also signposting people to become active within their communities.

You are likely to meet many people who have become experts in their long-term health condition or who have benefited from a statutory service and would like to share their experience and skills with their peers. Other people or services may have skills and assets that are not linked to a health need but can be used to benefit individuals and the wider community, raising health and well-being and reducing health inequalities and social deprivation. Statutory services can use social prescribing to refer people to these non-clinical services. Below is an overview of the types of asset-based activities that people can become involved in.

Peer interventions

Peer-based interventions are an effective way to engage people as they can improve communication and provide support to people who have a common understanding or experience of a health need. Peer supporters can be educated to engage effectively in community-based activities as an extension and enhancement of the statutory provision. These activities can range from one-to-one peer support to mentoring and education activities across a range of health needs, including peer smoking cessation, peer breastfeeding support, mental health peer support and supporting self-management of long-term conditions.

Health coaching and health trainers

We explored health coaching in Chapter 4; however, this can be delivered by a peer rather than a professional, including smoking cessation support or one-to-one diet and exercise management. Health trainers can work in a primary care team to enhance health provision.

Group activities

Many people prefer the support of a group-based activity as they feel the mental and physical benefits of a shared social activity. There are numerous community groups that provide support to their members, ranging from groups that focus on managing a health need, such as diet and exercise groups, to those that engage people to enjoy a social activity, such as gardening, painting or sport.

Volunteering

Many people will volunteer in their community, whether it be to support the local charity shop, become a befriender, join a 'good neighbour' scheme or engage in a community-wide activity. Community champions support their local community through the sharing of skills, knowledge and time to improve health and well-being and support local developments. Volunteering is an important community function as it promotes the health and well-being of the volunteer and those they are supporting. Participating in local volunteering activities can improve health equity between social groups (PHE, 2018b).

Viewing people as collaborators in care and service provision is an important change in the dynamic between health professionals and service users. With the increasing pressures on resources and the need to develop innovative ways of working, empowering communities and the people within them is a vital step towards sustainable service provision.

Chapter summary

This chapter has enabled you to develop an appreciation of how community empowerment can support sustainable provision of services at a time when there is significant pressure on resources. We have explored the various types of communities, as well as how marginalisation can adversely affect people's health and well-being.

We have considered asset-based approaches to community engagement and how people can be engaged within communities to improve health and well-being. Finally, we have considered how nurses and our multi-agency colleagues can work with people and communities to support innovative and sustainable service delivery.

Activities: Brief outline answers

Activity 6.1   Critical thinking (page 85)

These lists are not exhaustive:

- *Place-based*: Village (rural), island (e.g. Outer Hebrides), street, housing estate (council or privately owned), tower block, inner city, retirement complex, university campus.
- *Common identity*: Religious groups (e.g. Buddhist, Catholic, Church of England, Jehovah's Witness, Jewish, Muslim); cultural groups (e.g. Asian, Caribbean, Eastern European, Greek, travellers); occupational groups (this can be an extensive list of professions, and of course it includes nurses/student nurses, medical professionals, NHS staff, etc., but also groups without 'professional' status, such as volunteer groups, factory workers, sex workers, etc.); social groups (e.g. sports groups, health groups such as dieting clubs/walking groups, organised groups such as the Women's Institute, the Lions, the Freemasons, university societies, etc.); support/self-help/peer-led groups organised around a health need – these may be led by a charity or volunteer organisation, or they may be peer-led (e.g. diabetes, cancer support, stillbirth and neonatal death, private breastfeeding groups, mental health groups, learning disability groups); marginalised groups (e.g. sex workers, migrants/refugees/asylum seekers, travellers, LGBTQ+).
- *Locating information*: Many local council websites will host information on a range of groups available in the local area. The public health teams based in county councils will have a plan of improving health and well-being in their local community (including local project and initiatives), and these will be available on their websites. Many charity, sports and self-help/peer-led groups will also have their own websites or social media information.

Your exploration of a chosen community will be unique to you. You may need to consider whether they have any challenges accessing services and how these may be addressed. Are there any cultural, religious or linguistic considerations?

Activity 6.2 Reflection (page 86)

As a reflection, your answer will be highly personal to you. However, some common themes may be linked to the sense of support you gain from engaging with your university, local or national student groups. You may feel that the common anxieties and stresses of being a student nurse at your university are reduced by being able to chat to others in a similar position. Students may also engage in activities within specific nursing fields to raise the profile of their field. You may also be involved in community engagement activities (e.g. supporting widening participation initiatives as a student ambassador). Many students are active with unions, representing student nurses locally and nationally as a collective voice, particularly in raising the profile of key issues such as the financial challenges facing student nurses today.

Activity 6.3 Critical thinking (page 89)

Hopefully, you have been able to identify the public health strategy as a key element of the local authority's approach to reducing inequalities. There should also be policies and strategies that consider green spaces, local housing, infrastructure (roads, public transport and access) and economic developments (types of employment) within the area. The public-facing area of their website will also have a focus on community development, accessing resources and importantly how people can engage in developing services for their local community, whether this be place-based or group-based.

Activity 6.4 Leadership and management (page 97)

Exploring the local council website (including the public health team pages), the local community magazine and newspapers, as well as locating and following various support groups online and on social media, are some of the ways you can find out what is happening in your local area, as well as what activities may support your client population.

Building this knowledge into your daily practice is helpful when signposting people to services, activities and resources. You may even identify a service improvement development that involves collaboration with community groups and statutory services to meet the needs of the community with which you work.

Useful websites

www.instituteofhealthequity.org

The Institute of Health Equity is a leading source of current evidence in relation to inequalities in health.

www.kingsfund.org.uk

The King's Fund is a useful website to explore health topics and up-to-date perspectives on healthcare provision.

https://ukhsalibrary.koha-ptfs.co.uk/practice-examples/caba/

The UK Health Security Agency has listed examples (with links) to practice examples of community-centred asset-based initiatives.

Chapter 7

Health promotion at a population level

NMC Future Nurse: Standards of Proficiency for Registered Nurses

This chapter will address the following platforms and proficiencies:

Platform 1: Being an accountable professional

At the point of registration, the registered nurse will be able to:

1.13 demonstrate the skills and abilities required to develop, manage and maintain appropriate relationships with people, their families, carers and colleagues.

Platform 2: Promoting health and preventing ill health

At the point of registration, the registered nurse will be able to:

2.1 understand and apply the aims and principles of health promotion, protection and improvement and the prevention of ill health when engaging with people.

2.5 promote and improve mental, physical, behavioural and other health-related outcomes by understanding and explaining the principles, practice and evidence base for health screening programmes.

2.6 understand the importance of early years and childhood experiences and the possible impact on life choices, mental, physical and behavioural health and well-being.

2.7 understand and explain the contribution of social influences, health literacy, individual circumstances, behaviours and lifestyle choices to mental, physical and behavioural health outcomes.

2.11 promote health and prevent ill health by understanding and explaining to people the principles of pathogenesis, immunology and the evidence base for immunisation, vaccination and herd immunity.

Chapter aims

After reading this chapter, you will be able to:

- define population health promotion;
- describe the role of **public health surveillance** and the use of surveillance data to inform population health strategies, including the reduction of inequalities;
- discuss how health promotion at a population level involves strategic policy development, regulation and communication of health information;
- explore how nurses contribute to population health activities.

Case study: Owen

Owen is ten years old and lives in Cornwall. Owen's mum, Freya, is speaking to the school nurse about Owen's recent growth measurements taken at school by the school nursing team for the National Child Measurement Programme. She has received a letter to say that Owen is overweight and is at higher risk of health conditions as he gets older.

I am very upset that we received this letter. Owen is no different to the rest of the kids in his class. To say that he is overweight is nonsense, and to try to scare us that he will get health conditions like cancer and heart disease is just wrong. He has a healthy appetite and we eat plenty of fruit and vegetables every week. He is very active at school too.

Introduction

We have seen over the past three chapters that health promotion involves interventions with people, families and communities. Population health promotion is concerned with wider health and well-being needs at a population level. It involves wide-reaching policies and interventions to address health needs of populations as a whole. Public health specialists analyse data and provide advice on managing health needs at a population level. All nurses engage in public health activities to promote health and well-being to the people we provide services to. During your programme you will be engaged in public health activities, supporting people who access services, and may even contribute to evidence-based practice through the collection of public health surveillance data. If you are interested in advancing your future career in public health nursing, there are nurse specialist roles such as school nursing and health visiting.

The COVID-19 pandemic has focused everyone's attention on population health measures to reduce transmission of the virus, infection rates, long-term sequelae and deaths. However, it is important to not lose focus on long-standing population health needs that continue to have impacts for people's health and well-being. Key population health activities address health behaviours that have negative impacts on people's health, such as smoking, obesity, poor diet and alcohol misuse, which can lead to various health impacts such as heart disease and cancer.

Population health measures do not create a static situation where one intervention will be enough to improve the health of the majority of people in a population. Many of the influences on the health and well-being needs of individuals, families and communities are constantly changing. In addition to individual physical health needs and personal choices, there are social, environmental and economic factors continuously impacting on physical and mental health. These elements, coupled with political and legislative decisions at national and local government levels, influence people's health and well-being, as well as the provision and availability of resources within and across communities.

This chapter focuses on the aspects associated with promoting health at a population level. It will clarify how population health is defined and how agencies use public health surveillance to inform key population-wide strategies to address specific health needs. We will explore how surveillance data can provide a national and local focus on key determinants of health and well-being, as well as why reducing inequalities in health is so important. We will also consider how national government and local authorities, in consultation with key stakeholders, utilise the data from public health surveillance to address key health targets through strategic policies, legislation and population-level health promotion campaigns. Finally, we will explore how we, as nurses, are a key resource in the promotion of health at a population level.

What is population health?

There have been many moments in history that have evolved our understanding of the links between people's health and the various elements that impact on mortality and morbidity. John Snow's realisation that cholera was spreading from the Broad Street pump to the local community in London in 1854 is probably one of the most well known. Using simple data collection methods, he identified a causal link between the local water supply and the cases of cholera. Armed with this knowledge, he implemented a simple intervention in decommissioning the Broad Street water pump, which resulted in the outbreak being curtailed. This is an early example of using epidemiology to improve the health of people within a community.

Over time, the art and science of public health has become a key area in identifying and taking steps to manage the health of populations. The approach to public health has similarly evolved. Historically, public health focused on a utilitarian perspective, which embraced the notion that improving the health of people would reduce the individual's dependency on the state and increase employability and productivity. However, there is now the understanding that we live in an ever-changing environment where individual and population health is impacted by multiple elements, including climate change and limited natural resources. Therefore, sustainability of natural and physical resources is a necessary consideration in conjunction with the wider determinants of health to improve population health and well-being (Rayner and Lang, 2012).

Taking the various elements of population health into consideration, the King's Fund defines population health as:

> *An approach aimed at improving the health of an entire population. It is about improving the physical and mental health outcomes and well-being of people within and across a defined local, regional or national population, while reducing health inequalities. It includes action to reduce the occurrence of ill health, action to deliver appropriate health and care services and action on the wider determinants of health.*

(King's Fund, 2018a, p18)

Who is responsible for population health within the UK?

Within the UK, population health is the remit of public health departments embedded within national and local government. Each country that forms the UK has its own statutory departments of health and specific public health teams both at national and locality levels. These teams are based in local councils and work with other statutory bodies (such as the NHS, the police and state education providers) and allied organisations to develop and implement policies and frameworks to address the key needs of the people living within their jurisdictions. Nurses and other multi-professional workers are instrumental in implementing many of the population health approaches that are mandated by national and local authorities.

There are three main premises to public health:

1. the *prevention* of ill health through empowering people to adopt healthier behaviours;

2. the *protection* of the population through the surveillance of public health data, including communicable diseases, screening for disease and immunisation rates;

3. the *promotion* of health and well-being through education and providing/commissioning services to meet defined health needs.

From these overarching principles, public health departments are active on multiple levels, including policy development and taking action on health risks and emergencies. They closely monitor key indicators relating to health improvement, health protection, premature mortality and healthcare and the wider determinants of health. This enables the departments to define public health outcomes and population needs. These outcomes include ways to tackle inequalities that lead to socio-economic deprivation, and addressing policies, legislation and initiatives to reduce the contributing factors of mortality and morbidity, including those related to obesity, cancer and heart disease. Another activity is to provide data analysis through public health surveillance to support governmental policies and actions. These will include disease statistics, deprivation analyses and the multiple elements that contribute to the wider determinants of health. Finally, they also conduct surveillance of communicable and non-communicable diseases, as well as screening and vaccination rates.

Understanding the health needs of the population: the importance of data

Epidemiology is the scientific approach to studying and analysing health data to identify key trends in health and disease and subsequently informs policy and practice. This scientific approach is important to track the influence of health behaviours and conditions that have a significant impact on population health and well-being.

The National Child Measurement Programme (NHS Digital, 2021a) is one example of a national data collection activity that is analysed by epidemiologists. It provides vital scientific data regarding the obesity trends among school-age children, as well as an indicator as to whether interventions are being effective. The data collection is usually undertaken by school nursing teams. The data supports our evidence-based practice, enabling engagement with parents and children to raise awareness and begin actions to address childhood obesity and reducing the potential risk of associated health conditions that impact individuals in adulthood. However, for parents receiving information that their child is overweight or obese can be challenging, and for some parents it can feel that their parenting is being questioned. This is when our communication skills are vital in maintaining a supportive and empowering approach to effectively engage with parents and children (PHE, 2019a).

Identifying population health needs requires the gathering of intelligence to inform necessary actions to address population health. Key to this approach is the gathering of public health surveillance data. Public health surveillance is the systematic collection of multiple sources of information, which are subsequently analysed and interpreted, and which then form the foundation of strategies that aim to address population health needs.

The data that contribute to public health surveillance derive from many different sources. There are rules imposed to ensure the data are collected so that they are accurate and reliable, enabling robust analysis to take place. The data are then presented as 'national data' within the official public health **data sets**.

There are formal routes for collecting the data and several agencies may be involved, including statutory and external agencies (e.g. NHS, local authorities, external organisations such as Cancer Research UK or the British Heart Foundation). The collected data cover a wide range of information, such as use of health services, disease statistics, census data, local and national health profiles, inequalities and socio-economic deprivation.

Our role in population-level data

We all contribute to data used for population-level health surveillance every day of our lives, but most of the time we are oblivious to this happening unless we are completing a census or survey. Most of our activities and use of services add to these data, whether it is our occupation and work-related health, our use of services, including the NHS, our consumer choices, or our housing and living conditions.

While we contribute to data, as nurses we also collect data, although you may not be aware you are doing so. When you are working within the clinical environment, you are collecting data every time you write in an online patient health record, complete an incident report or refer a person to another service. Hidden behind computerised heathcare record systems are a series of complex data codes that relate to your activities with the person, such as pressure area care, whether a new mother is breastfeeding or whether a person was referred to social care. So, accurate recording in healthcare records is essential to both the safety and ongoing care of people, as well as in the collection of health surveillance data.

Interpreting public health surveillance data to inform population health strategies

Public health surveillance data enable ongoing monitoring of particular aspects of population health protection, promotion and prevention. The data enable subsequent policies and interventions to be evaluated to understand their impact in order to develop future strategies. There are official departments in each of the countries which form the United Kingdom that are responsible for public health surveillance in their populations. In England in 2021, the UK Government restructured Public Health England, which was the government agency responsible for this surveillance in England, into two distinct agencies. The UK Health Security Agency (UKHSA) is responsible for health surveillance and national response relating to communicable diseases and health hazards. This includes monitoring data on immunisations, a range of infectious diseases and emerging outbreaks, infections acquired in healthcare and chemical and environmental hazards. The Office for Health Improvement and Disparities (OHID) is responsible for health prevention and inequalities, public health surveillance of non-communicable diseases and the analysis, management and leadership of national public health data. There is a Chief Public Health Nurse who is responsible for national leadership of public health activities within nursing, midwifery and allied health services.

The data collated by the national agencies is used to inform whether there needs to be a regional, local or national response to the health need, as well as whether this response requires urgent action (in the case of disease outbreak such as we have seen with COVID-19) or planned action that addresses outcomes in a long-term sustained way (e.g. key health promotion targets such as smoking cessation and obesity).

Communicable diseases: the case of measles

Cases of highly contagious diseases such as measles, rubella and meningitis are 'notifiable diseases' and medical practitioners have a statutory duty to report suspected cases. Rapid mobilisation of public health protection responses to outbreaks of notifiable diseases is essential to swiftly implement strategies to contain the spread in order to protect the wider population, as well as supporting services to manage such cases.

Eradication of measles is an international and national target (WHO, 2020). The national data for vaccination and communicable disease rates are analysed within the UK continuously, so there are data sets covering several years. The national data contribute to the WHO's measles eradication global data. In 2015, the low levels of measles cases recorded led to the UK receiving measles eradication status.

However, globally, there have been challenges in maintaining effective levels of vaccinated individuals, exacerbated by growing numbers of people who do not believe in vaccinations for their children, as well as the physical movement of unvaccinated people across borders through planned and forced migration. As we discussed in Chapter 5, there are specific challenges within the UK relating to low rates of vaccinations in some communities. The reduction in vaccination rates of measles prevents herd immunity, leading to more measles outbreaks and placing those who are vulnerable and unable to have immunisation at greater risk. In 2019, the UK lost its measles eradication status following increased numbers of measles outbreaks (UK Health Security Agency, 2019b).

Activity 7.1 will enable you to explore the debate that has surrounded the national approach to measles vaccinations.

Activity 7.1 Critical thinking

Read 'Should Measles Vaccination Be Compulsory?' (Draeger et al., 2019) (for the link, see the further reading section at the end of this chapter). Read the article in two sections.

First, read Draeger's comments. What evidence supports the rationale that Draeger gives for their stance? Do you agree with these comments?

Then read Bedford and Elliman's response. What evidence do the two authors give for their stance? Has this altered your thoughts following your initial reading of Draeger's comments?

An outline answer is provided at the end of the chapter.

Hopefully, this activity raised your awareness of the various elements that need to be carefully considered before changes to policy and potential legislation occur. As nurses it is imperative that we understand debates on key topics to enhance our delivery of evidence-based practice. We may even collectively contribute to these debates through our practice networks, or individually contribute where we have specialist knowledge.

In 2019, the public health response to the loss of measles eradication status included increasing population awareness through wide media coverage, targeted information to sectors of the population (including parents of young children and university students), reviewing service provision and providing resources for health professionals to support conversations with people to provide consistent messages.

Health surveillance and the wider determinants of health

At a population level, there are social, economic and environmental factors that are commonly termed the 'wider determinants of health'. These determinants relate to factors that are external to the individual and family but have a significant impact on everyday life. Indicators such as employment, income and work conditions, the natural environment, housing, healthcare services, access to clean water and sanitation and agriculture and food production all contribute to the wider determinants of health (Rayner and Lang, 2012). Proactively addressing these determinants such as improving employment prospects, or ensuring health services are tailored to improve access, can have a positive impact on health and well-being.

Health surveillance data of the wider determinants of health indicators are important as they reflect the levels of health and well-being in the population as a whole and within localities. Higher rates of crime and unemployment, poor-quality education and employment and poor access and quality within the natural and built environment (housing and access to green spaces) can contribute to, and have a negative impact on, health and well-being, leading to inequalities in health, socio-economic deprivation and poorer health outcomes for people (OHID, 2022b).

Exploring the wider determinants of health data

There are data sets produced within the Government public health departments in England, Northern Ireland, Scotland and Wales. A resource for this part of the chapter is the Office for Health Improvement and Disparities fingertip tool, which explores the wider determinants of health data in England (OHID, 2022b). Becoming familiar with data tools and navigating your way around these resources will be an important aspect of your evidence-based practice. By critically exploring the data, you will develop an awareness of how data and statistics can influence policies and legislation both nationally and locally. These policies aim to have a positive impact on the local population through the effective provision of services, including housing, employment, welfare and health.

The wider determinants of health data provide information on key categories of wider determinants in localities within the UK, enabling comparison of these data with other localities. This provides a visualisation of where there are localities in greater need, as well as monitoring existing inequalities within and between localities. Furthermore, where localities have received funding and interventions to address a need, the data contribute to the overall evaluation.

Using data to improve your knowledge of local and national population health

Reading and interpreting data is a skill that you will gradually develop throughout your pre-registration nurse education and throughout your career. It is important to develop your critical awareness of how data inform policy and practice.

Of course, the way data are used can be dependent on the purpose of the organisation that is using them. Indeed, data can be manipulated to provide a sensationalist headline in the media or to underline a political statement. Therefore, being critically aware also requires a level of questioning of what the data mean, what the 'agenda' of the publisher is and whether the findings reflect the true picture.

By developing your skills in exploring the data, you will have a critical appreciation of the information, as well as how it is relevant to your scope of practice and the local population. Nurses use health surveillance data in conjunction with other evidence to inform their practice and raise awareness within their organisation of the needs of the local population. They will also use data to act as a catalyst to work with other stakeholders and service users to campaign and lobby for change or the implementation of innovations in services both locally and nationally.

Activity 7.2 enables you to develop your skills in exploring the OHID wider determinants of health data sets.

Activity 7.2   Evidence-based practice and research

Using the internet, access the OHID 'fingertip' resource data set on the wider determinants of health using the link in the 'useful websites' section at the end of this chapter.

Take time to explore the functions within each section of the data sets by clicking different tabs and drop-down boxes, as well as changing how you 'view' the data. You can click on the different options to see the data presented in table and graph form. Each key indicator within the data set is categorised into subsets of data. By clicking on the downward arrow in the 'key indicator' function box, you can view these subsets.

Choose one particular topic within one of the key indicator sections that interests you. Compare different localities across England. What do you notice about the variations in data across England? Are there any variations within neighbouring, or northern and southern, England localities? Why do you think these variations exist?

Your exploration of the data set will be unique to you; therefore, there is no outline answer at the end of the chapter.

Your interaction with Activity 7.2 will be unique to you; however, you may have noticed that there were certain 'trends' in the data. For example, some localities have lower unemployment, higher educational attainment and improved access to resources compared to other localities who have consistently poorer outcomes. Critically exploring the data requires a curiosity about what may be influencing the data and the experiences of people within the localities.

Population health professionals and government organisations will use health data in various ways to articulate how the data is relevant to populations in regional and national contexts and to inform policies. They may present statistical data in different formats to provide accessible ways to visualise the regional variations. One such source is the Annual Fuel Poverty statistics in England, 2022 and the handy fact sheet which provides an overview of the data (Department for Business, Energy and Industrial Strategy (BEIS), 2022). Fuel poverty impacts people significantly and cold housing presents a risk to health and contributes to winter deaths (Marmot, 2010).

Activity 7.3   Critical thinking

You can use your newly gained knowledge to begin to explore the data that are presented within the fuel poverty data sheet and develop your critical awareness of potential issues for the people living in different regions in England.

Read the BEIS factsheet on fuel poverty. There is a link provided at the end of the chapter in the useful websites section.

As you read through the information, consider the different ways data is presented. To critically explore this information ask yourself a series of questions:

- What do you understand about the information presented?
- What might be influencing the data?
- While the data focuses on energy efficiency, energy prices and incomes, what other wider determinants of health may help you as a nurse to understand the experiences of people living in the different locations in England?

To answer this question, you will need to think about *when* the data was collected, and *where* people live. You can also use the OHID 'fingertip' tool (see Activity 7.2) to look at various data relating to wider determinants of health in different areas of England.

An outline answer is provided at the end of this chapter.

One element you may have focused on is the difference between the geographical areas in England. Just a simple glance at the maps on page 3 of the fact sheet shows that the localities within the northern part of the UK have higher rates of fuel poverty than the localities in the south. Some of the localities with high fuel poverty are in mixed rural and urbanised areas, whereas others are in highly urbanised areas. People living in these areas may be affected by higher rates of socio-economic deprivation and unemployment.

You may be curious as to why fuel poverty and employment data are important in population health. In fact, in the UK, fuel poverty is now measured under the 'Low Income Low Energy Efficiency (LILEE)' metric which takes into consideration household income and energy efficiency of homes. From a health promotion perspective, when we consider the wider determinants of health, we can appreciate that people who may be living with limited access to money to afford adequate heating, or to make necessary energy efficiency changes to their homes, are more likely to need support with food and health needs too. Households may be fuel-poor due to low income, high fuel costs or living in poorly built housing. Importantly, fuel poverty has a particularly negative impact on vulnerable sectors of the population, including families with young children, older people and people with disabilities (Marmot et al., 2018). Having knowledge and understanding of the challenges that affect people within the communities where you also live and work will help you to consider the health and well-being needs of people you will provide services to.

Inequality of access to basic resources, employment and income contributes to socio-economic deprivation and inequalities in health. As we identified in the previous chapters, socio-economic deprivation and inequalities in health have an adverse impact on people's physical and mental well-being, as well as presenting a key concern for population health (Marmot, 2010).

Inequalities in health and the social divide: the impact on population health and well-being

> *Health inequalities go against the principles of social justice because they are avoidable. They do not occur randomly or by chance. They are socially determined by circumstances largely beyond an individual's control. These circumstances disadvantage people and limit their chance to live longer, healthier lives.*

> (NHS Health Scotland, 2019)

Over the past 40 years, there have been key reports that have shaped our understanding of the nation's health:

* the Black Report (DHSS, 1980);
* the Acheson Report (DH, 1998);
* the Marmot Review (Marmot, 2010).

These three key reports continued to highlight the impact of socio-economic deprivation, poverty and inequalities on sectors of the population. They also underlined the complexities of addressing population health and well-being, as well as the importance of continued efforts at political, organisational and societal levels to address individual, family and community health. Since the COVID-19 pandemic, new data has identified an increase in socio-economic deprivation and poverty, leading to renewed calls for the UK Government to support those in greater need (Marmot et al, 2020).

There are various types of inequalities experienced by people that influence socio-economic deprivation, whether it be income, employment, power or poverty, and all these contribute to inequalities in health. These inequalities are related to each other as people with lower incomes or who are unemployed, or working in low-paid, low-quality jobs, may also be living in poverty. Furthermore, people from lower socio-economic groups may feel powerless within their communities, and this makes it harder for them to access services and resources or challenge social norms. The country's taxation and benefit system may also have a negative impact on household incomes. It is important not to assume that people who are in employment are not in poverty as the household income may not meet their needs. A continuing concern within the UK today is that there are still people, particularly families with children, who are living in poverty. Current statistics identify that in the UK, 14.5 million people are living in poverty, of which 4.3 million are children. Significantly the welfare system, which sets levels of benefit payments, has contributed to this figure, and more people in employment are living in poverty where their income does not meet living costs (Joseph Rowntree Foundation, 2022).

Impact of inequalities

As we have explored in previous chapters, the impact of inequalities on people is significant. Mental and physical health and well-being are affected by inequalities in health and socio-economic deprivation. People who live in localities that have higher rates of deprivation and in lower socio-economic groups have poorer health outcomes, whether this be premature mortality or living in poor health in later years (Roberts and Bell, 2015; Steel et al., 2018). It is a legal requirement for statutory bodies to collaborate to ensure that reducing inequalities is an integral element of their work and policies (Health and Care Act, 2022).

Nevertheless, national data analysis continues to demonstrate a social divide between the least and most deprived sectors of the population. To evidence this, we can return to Owen's case study at the beginning of this chapter. The National Child Measurement Programme population-level data of children in Owen's age group (Year 6, age 10–11) indicate a social gradient influencing obesity rates, with the most deprived areas recording significantly higher rates than in the least deprived areas (see Figure 7.1).

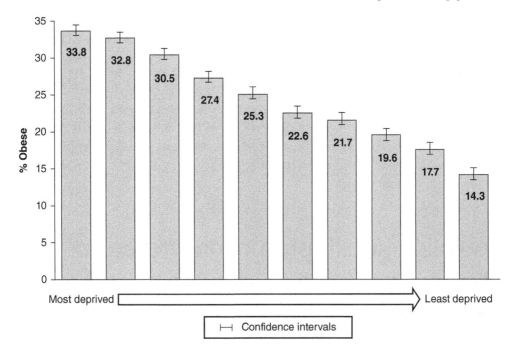

Figure 7.1 National Child Measurement Programme, England 2020/21 school year, Year 6: levels of obesity and deprivation data based on Index of Multiple Deprivation deciles (child's postcode) (NHS Digital, 2021)

More importantly, despite various interventions to reduce childhood obesity locally and nationally over several years, the data demonstrate that the gap between the least and most deprived areas has increased over time. While in the least deprived areas obesity rates remained similar, in the most deprived areas the rates increased (see Figure 7.2).

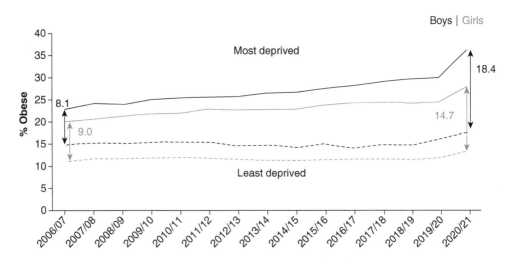

Figure 7.2 National Child Measurement Programme 2020–2021, deprivation data showing the gap between the most and least deprived and sex of child (NHS Digital, 2021b)

The causative factors are complex and are influenced by multiple elements, including health behaviours, availability and choice of food and drinks, the family's approach to physical activity and wider influences involving social, economic and political factors.

From a population health perspective, addressing health issues such as childhood obesity is important as it has implications for the individual throughout their lifespan and increases the risk of other health conditions such as type 2 diabetes, heart disease and cancers. Public health strategies to reduce health risks and promote health and well-being require multilevel approaches, including policies, regulation and effective use of health promotion campaigns.

Population health promotion strategies: policy implementation, regulation and health campaigns

Defining population health needs and implementing outcomes requires multilevel actions to address the key determinants of health and well-being. Strategic policies will identify actions to address the key target and identify desired outcomes. Regulation and taxation may be enforced on several elements that encompass sectors of industry and provision of services including elements that impact on the environment, food production and advertising, housing, infrastructure and employment in order to address causative factors, encourage behaviour change and improve conditions. Public health campaigns address health education and health behaviour change. These can be targeted at a sector of the population (e.g. promoting screening programmes to a target group such as prostate cancer in men) or a whole population via a mass media campaign (e.g. smoking cessation).

Strategic policies

As we have seen, health surveillance data increase understanding of the health needs of the population. This needs to be developed into a coherent strategy in order to mobilise effective policy implementation across all sectors.

Wide consultation enables clarification and focus, and involves organisations, groups and individuals with specialist and expert status (including service user groups) to contribute to the in-depth exploration of the public health issue. This ensures that the impact of any proposed strategy has been thoroughly considered.

Nurses and nursing organisations, such as the Royal College of Nursing (RCN), are actively engaged in consultations that relate to nursing and population health. Part of this role may encompass acting as expert advisers, representing the interests of the profession, and importantly advocating for and supporting people in the target population who may not have a strong voice. This is particularly important for people who are powerless and vulnerable, including those living in poverty, who have disabilities or who derive from marginalised communities.

This does not mean that developing and implementing health policies is straight-forward or swift. Some population health changes can take a long time to agree and enact policies, as well as see desired health benefits. Sometimes the competing inter-ests of key stakeholders can slow or even derail intended population health changes. Smoking laws and related policies are a clear example of this. In the twentieth century, the tobacco industry was powerful and influential, and engaged in tactics to undermine and adversely influence attempts to address the growing concerns about the adverse health impacts of tobacco smoking for millions of people across the world. Despite the significant body of evidence linking tobacco smoke and poor health outcomes, it took over 50 years to implement the smoking ban in the UK (Rayner and Lang, 2012).

Ethical implications of population health actions

It is worth discussing at this point the ethical dimensions of population health approaches. *Non-maleficence* is the principle of doing no harm; therefore, public health policies need to ensure that people are not harmed by any intervention or regulation. Indeed, the collec-tion of health surveillance data and research is guided by strict ethical and legal principles.

We have already highlighted the legal requirement for health and social care sectors to address health and well-being and reduce inequalities. This relates to the ethical notion of *justice* and includes *beneficence*. Reducing the challenges and impact of health inequalities promotes equity, reflecting the intention to enable everyone to experience good levels of health and well-being, and needs to be achieved through social, eco-nomic, environmental and health actions.

Implementation of legislation and regulations can encroach on people's *right to autonomy*. Legislation, such as the seatbelt law, laws criminalising illicit drug use, implementation of laws relating to tobacco restrictions, and more recently the imple-mentation of taxes and advertising restrictions to reduce obesity, reduces individual autonomy and free will (Coggon and Adams, 2021). However, the legislation has been implemented for the 'greater good' and based on clear evidence, and therefore encompasses the ethical principle of *beneficence*.

Regulating for population health

Many regulations address the wider determinants of health and are aimed at public and private sector organisations, such as manufacturers, the housing sector, farming and food production and media and advertising.

Regulations are also integral to targeted health promotion actions. In the case of tobacco smoking, there has been a multifaceted approach to addressing the elements associated with tobacco use. These approaches have aimed to remove or reframe the physical, social and environmental elements that influence people's cues to smoking. These include banning smoking in public places, advertising restrictions and age limitations on the purchase of tobacco products.

These legislative actions have been in addition to the increase in smoking cessation services, offering people a variety of opportunities to address their smoking habit. Using behaviour change and empowerment approaches, NHS services provide a range of person-centred options to support smoking cessation (Better Health, 2022).

Public health campaigns

While regulatory and strategic policy implementation is important, an essential step in addressing population health needs is the engagement of the target audience through structured health promotion campaigns.

Communicating health messages requires a clear understanding of the health issue and the most effective way to inform and engage people in the target population. There are many methods of promoting health with people using focused health promotion materials. You may have seen leaflets and posters in GP surgeries, public toilets and in the clinical areas while on placement covering a range of health topics and targeting a diverse range of population groups. You will also be involved in promoting health messages and working with people in various health promotion activities within your clinical practice.

If the health need impacts a large portion of the population, then a wider, co-ordinated approach is necessary. This is when mass media campaigns will be used to communicate the health promotion message on multiple media platforms to reach a wide audience.

There are many national campaigns designed to address the health needs of people within the population and engage a wide range of media in which to do so.

In Activity 7.4, you will explore a well-known mass media campaign to look at how they engage with their target population.

Activity 7.4   Critical thinking

Locate the Better Health – Healthier Families media materials via their website (Better Health – Healthier Families, 2022). (See useful websites section at the end of this chapter.)

What is the range of materials used to promote the health message? Who is the intended target audience? How have they communicated their message visually, in the images used and the information that is given? Do you think it meets the needs of the target audience? Is it accessible to a range of people within the target audience? Is there anything you would change to make it more accessible, and why?

An outline answer is provided at the end of the chapter.

This activity has enabled you to consider how health messages can be communicated in different ways to the target audience. Public health campaigns will take different approaches to communicating their key messages based on social marketing approaches which use elements of commercial marketing techniques, social psychology, behaviour change theory and empowerment concepts to educate the target audience, empower people to take action and promote behaviour change (Rayner and Lang, 2012).

The role of the nurse in population health

There are nurses who have a particular responsibility and specialist education to deliver public health activities within their daily nurse role. These nurses lead on key public health initiatives such as:

- implementation of the Healthy Child Programme and working closely with families and communities to reduce inequalities (health visitor and school nurses);
- carrying out the National Child Measurement Programme and HPV immunisation campaign (school nurse);
- monitoring of occupational hazards as part of an employer's legal duty (occupational health nurse).

Other nursing roles undertake key activities that promote health and well-being, collecting health surveillance data, including immunisation rates, screening and the monitoring of specific health conditions. They may be general practice nurses or nurse specialists in a wide range of health conditions.

You too will have an essential role in health promotion and engaging in population health activities, as reflected in *Future Nurse: Standards of Proficiency for Registered Nurses* (NMC, 2018a). Your pre-registration nursing programme will prepare you for your role in health promotion to support people with whatever health need matters to them and deliver brief interventions with people and families. Keeping up to date with the current health and well-being needs of the population will also enable you to translate this to your sphere of nursing. As a qualified nurse, you will develop an in-depth understanding of the people you work with, the impact of their health needs and the challenges and benefits of living and working in the locality in which they live. This will enable you to advocate for the vulnerable and work closely with people and groups to collaborate and empower them to raise the profile of their health and well-being needs within their local area.

Finally, being active within nursing forums will enable you to actively contribute to consultations on population health strategies and policies.

Chapter summary

This chapter has explored the promotion of health and well-being at a population level. We have considered the role of public health departments, as well as how health surveillance

(Continued)

(Continued)

shapes our understanding of the needs of the population to enable national and local government to set key population health strategic objectives. We have enabled you to explore
health surveillance data in order to highlight the importance of developing your awareness
of this evidence and its use within your practice. Finally, we have considered how population
health targets are addressed through a multifaceted approach that includes developing strategic policies, implementation of regulation and health promotion campaigns.

Activities: Brief outline answers

Activity 7.1   Critical thinking (page 107)

Both sets of authors make compelling arguments. When reading this information, it is important
to be critical about the statements being made. Are the statistics correct? If you are not sure, then
access the vaccination rates as published by the relevant public health department for the country
you live in. Consider whether the countries that Draeger highlights are comparable to the UK perspective. What impact would legislation have on all sectors of the population? Bedford and Elliman
take an objective stance, looking at causative factors that are influencing the drop in uptake rather
than presenting parents as the problem. Do you agree with them? Finally, it would be important to
reflect on how the authors' competing interests impact their particular stance.

Activity 7.3   Critical thinking (page 110)

The fuel poverty fact sheet helps us to understand how different elements may impact individuals, but the data is presented from a business perspective using the Low Income Low Energy
Efficiency Metric to calculate the data and lacks the person-centred element that we will need as
nurses to understand the experiences of people who we care for. Be aware that fact sheets con-
dense information into 'bite size' but this will often miss out explanatory detail, so you should
also get used to locating the full reports to widen your knowledge. Looking at the fact sheet,
you will see that the data is from 2020, so data will be affected by the pandemic and will include
the loss of income many people experienced, impacting on available income for household
costs, such as heating, home repairs and buying food and clothing. Location is another element.
Those people living in northern areas of England will experience colder weather, meaning costs
to heat homes will be higher than in southern areas. Also, rural areas may have poorer transport
infrastructures which may impact on availability of fuel sources. Finally, population demographics will also influence the experience of people living in fuel poverty. Areas with high densities of
deprivation and poverty will increase the numbers of people living in fuel poverty.

Activity 7.4   Critical thinking (page 116)

The Better Health – Healthier Families campaigns approach communicating the health message
in very different ways.

The materials use imagery, colours and resources which are bright and vibrant and clearly targeted at children and parents. There is a diverse range of images of people to engage with a
wide range of people within the population. The messages are conveyed in positive, empowering
terminology.

The campaign has developed a variety of resources, including mobile apps, to support people to
actively engage with the activities.

Further Reading

To assist you in engaging with Activity 7.1, access the article here:

Draeger et al. (2019) Should Measles Vaccination Be Compulsory? *British Medical Journal*, 365: 12359. Available at: **https://doi.org/10.1136/bmj.l2359**

Useful websites

https://assets.publishing.service.gov.uk/government/uploads/system/uploads/attachment_data/file/1056842/fuel-poverty-factsheet-2020.pdf

To assist your explorations in Activity 7.3, access the UK Government's fuel poverty fact sheet.

https://fingertips.phe.org.uk/profile/wider-determinants

To assist you in engaging with Activity 7.2, access the Office for Health Improvement and Disparities fingertip tool.

www.gov.uk/government/publications/commissioning-of-public-health-services-for-children/health-visiting-and-school-nursing-service-delivery-model#public-health-nurses-leading-the-healthy-child-programme

The UK Government updated the health visiting and school nurse model in 2021. This resource can assist you in understanding how nurses have a vital role in providing public health services for children, young people and their families.

www.kingsfund.org.uk/publications/health-and-care-act-key-questions

The King's Fund is a key source of information on a wider range of health and social care topics. This resource is useful to understand the new Health and Care Act that came into legislation in 2022.

Chapter 8 Promoting health in diverse and vulnerable populations

Platform 3: Assessing needs and planning care

At the point of registration, the registered nurse will be able to:

3.4   understand and apply a person-centred approach to nursing care, demonstrating shared assessment, planning, decision making and goal setting when working with people, their families, communities and populations of all ages.

3.9   recognise and assess people at risk of harm and the situations that may put them at risk, ensuring prompt action is taken to safeguard those who are vulnerable.

Platform 4: Providing and evaluating care

At the point of registration, the registered nurse will be able to:

4.2   work in partnership with people to encourage shared decision making in order to support individuals, their families and carers to manage their own care when appropriate.

Platform 6: Improving safety and quality of care

At the point of registration, the registered nurse will be able to:

6.11   acknowledge the need to accept and manage uncertainty and demonstrate an understanding of strategies that develop resilience in self and others.

Platform 7: Co-ordinating care

At the point of registration, the registered nurse will be able to:

7.9   facilitate equitable access to healthcare for people who are vulnerable or have a disability, demonstrate the ability to advocate on their behalf when required, and make necessary reasonable adjustments to the assessment, planning and delivery of their care.

Chapter aims

After reading this chapter, you will be able to:

- describe health concerns and issues of diverse and vulnerable populations;
- discuss selected cultural factors that may have an impact on the health and well-being of these groups;
- describe initiatives to address the health concerns of diverse and vulnerable groups of people.

Introduction

As nurses, we will be working with many different people, and we must treat them as individuals, and not treat them any differently to people who are similar to ourselves. The following chapter looks at the health promotion needs of emerging populations, diverse communities and vulnerable peoples. It seeks to understand the cultural diversity within society and the concerns and issues of emerging and vulnerable populations. It will discuss selected cultural factors that may have an impact on the health and well-being of emerging populations, before going on to explain strategies that the nurse could employ to meet the needs of individuals from a range of diverse backgrounds. The chapter will also allow you to examine your own beliefs and attitudes towards people from differing cultural and ethnic backgrounds. Finally, it will describe initiatives to address the healthcare concerns of emerging and vulnerable populations.

Case study: Amir and Kamilah Al-Ghazzawi

Amir and Kamilah Al-Ghazzawi have four children: Nirman (6 months), Julia (18 months), Hady (4 years) and Jamella (6 years). Amir is a land worker who immigrated to the UK four years ago. Kamilah is a homemaker who enjoys needlecraft and working with her hands. Amir and Kamilah have been asked to attend clinic and have their children vaccinated as part of the MMR vaccination programme, something that was not accessible to them in their **country of origin** but is promoted in the UK. MMR is a safe and effective combined vaccine that protects against three separate illnesses – measles, mumps and rubella – in a single injection. The full course of MMR vaccination requires two doses. The MMR vaccination is routinely given to children in the UK as part of the NHS childhood immunisation programme. The first dose of the MMR vaccine is offered to all babies at 1 year old. Children are given a second dose of the MMR before they start school, usually at 3 years and 4 months, although the second dose can be given as quickly as three months after the first if there's an urgent need, such as during an outbreak.

While sitting in the waiting room of the clinic, Amir and Kamilah can be heard arguing in a foreign language (Arabic). The receptionist tries to console them, but they seem very upset over something. The nurse intervenes, and together with the receptionist they try to get to the bottom of what is upsetting Amir and Kamilah. Kamilah, it seems, understands little English and communicates through her husband, who in turn has limited English and is unfamiliar with medical terminology. Both Amir and Kamilah do not understand what the injection is for and are frightened that it is going to make their children ill. The eldest child, Jamella, does not like needles and is also fearful of the injection and what might happen to her, and has started to cry. Neither Amir nor Kamilah understand their legal rights and whether they can refuse the injection. They are deeply worried that by refusing to allow their children the vaccination, they will have broken UK law and could be 'forcibly removed from this country' (this is not the case). The whole family are clearly upset and frightened about what is going to happen and feel, rightly or wrongly, that they do not have a choice in the matter.

Most developed countries, including the UK, do not have compulsory immunisation requirements, but instead issue recommendations, expecting parents to make an informed, autonomous (i.e. empowered) decision regarding their children's future well-being.

The increasing population of immigrants and the migration of people in search of work, housing and better living conditions has been a significant contributor to the presence of increasing numbers of major ethnic groups in the UK. The concept behind immigration and migration health encompasses the idea that there are various factors and conditions which influence health in certain groups of people, and we need to be aware of this as promoters of health.

Lifestyle and behaviour are central to the acquisition and development of major chronic diseases. To influence lifestyle and behaviour, health promoters must take into account the values, attitudes, culture and life circumstances of the individual. The nurses and staff in the case study above had difficulty communicating with the family and understanding the concerns of Amir and Kamilah and their children. Amir and Kamilah did not understand what was being asked of them, nor of their rights under English law, and were unsure of their status as immigrants to the UK.

Nurses need to actively embrace strategies to improve individual and population health outcomes and reduce health and other disparities. Effective strategies include a focus on the broad range of factors and conditions that have a strong influence on health, advocacy directed at reducing barriers to improved population health and engagement in policy making.

Understanding the needs of diverse and vulnerable populations can improve healthcare delivery by helping to focus resources such as screening programmes, education, resource allocation and help tailor health promotion activity to specific groups with specific needs. This requires diverse communities having equal access to services and information. Improved access for such populations might require provision of bilingual/bicultural staff; foreign language interpreting services; link workers/advocates; materials developed and tested for specific cultural, ethnic and linguistic groups; and translation services. Health messages should be tailored to reflect cultural drivers of behaviour that will increase knowledge using accessible language and including content that reflects the social norms and identity of the target community to increase engagement and awareness of the health risk and health promotion activities.

> ### Concept summary: What is meant by the terms 'immigrant', 'migrant', 'refugee' and 'asylum seeker'?
>
> Confusion remains as to the differences between the terms 'immigrant', 'migrant', 'refugee' and 'asylum seeker'. This situation is not helped by the way in which people use these terms, which can be heavily stigmatising.
>
> An immigrant is someone who makes a conscious decision to leave his or her home and move to a foreign country with the intention of settling there. Immigration generally falls under four major categories: family-based immigration (moving to be with closely related persons already living in the UK), employment-based immigration (skilled workers and business people), refugees and asylum seekers (people who are escaping persecution, torture or cruel and unusual punishment) and humanitarian immigration (people accepted as immigrants for humanitarian or compassionate reasons).
>
> A migrant is someone who is moving from place to place (within his or her own country or across borders), usually for economic reasons such as seasonal work. Similar to immigrants, migrants move in order to seek better opportunities for themselves or their families.
>
> A refugee is someone who, having escaped a country, has been granted legal status to stay in this country, whereas an asylum seeker is someone who is seeking protection from the dangers in his or her own country, but whose claim for refugee status has not been determined legally.
>
> (adapted from IRC, 2018)

Conditions surrounding the migration process can increase the vulnerability to ill health. Depending upon where the person comes from, there can be differences in the disease profiles and health risk factors between migrant and host populations, or inequalities in the access/uptake of preventative treatment outcomes. This is particularly true for those who migrate involuntarily, fleeing natural or man-made disasters. Migration also cuts across economic and social policies, human rights and equity issues, development agendas and social norms – all of which are relevant to migration health (Migration Data Portal, 2019).

Ethnicity, race and culture

Most health issues concern us equally, but some of our differences as individuals have implications for our health and well-being. These health-related differences between individuals and groups can be biological or cultural (e.g. sickle-cell anaemia is more common in black African populations). If we are to start to achieve changes in the health status of minority populations, health professionals and nurses must first understand the extraordinary diversity of the UK's population. This is an incredibly complex issue, and one open to misunderstanding. To start this process, we are going to look at what is meant by the terms 'ethnicity', 'race' and 'culture'. All three terms figure largely in the literature and are subject to legal definition and action.

An ethnic group or ethnicity is a population group whose members identify with each other on the basis of common nationality or shared cultural traditions. Hutchinson and Smith (1996) defined an ethnic group, or *ethnie*, as consisting of six characteristics, including a name for the group, common ancestry, historical memories, elements of common culture, a common language and a link with a homeland; however, they did note that the presence of all six features is not critical for an ethnic group to exist. Some ethnic groups also share linguistic or religious traits, while others share a common group history but not a common language or religion.

Race

The terms 'ethnicity' and 'race' are sometimes confused, and while they are different, they are also somewhat alike. A person's race has been defined as *a dynamic set of historically derived and initialised ideas and practices that sorts people into ethnic groups according to perceived physical and behavioural human characteristics* (Markus, 2006, page 654). Most people think of race in biological terms, although the term has been used for political means in order to justify some action, often exploitation, of one group of people by another. A minority group consists of people who are living within a society in which they are usually disadvantaged in relation to power, control of their own lives and wealth.

Culture

Cultures are said to consist of *systems of shared ideas and rules and meanings that underlie and are expressed in the ways that human beings live* within groups of people often from the same country or region (Matsumoto, 1996, page 16). They are a set of guidelines (both implicit and explicit) that individuals inherit as members of a particular society, which tell them how to view the world, how to experience it emotionally and how to behave in it in relation to other people and to the natural environment (Holland and Hogg, 2010). Careful consideration needs to be given so as not to confuse 'ethnicity' and 'nationality', but to ask the person how they identify themselves and their needs. You may wish to explore your culture in Activity 8.1.

Activity 8.1   Reflection

Cultures differ from one another in the ways they view the world. You are not born with culture. Culture is learned, first in the family, then in school, then in the community and other social organisations such as the Church (Purnell, 2002).

If we stop to consider it, the great majority of our conscious behaviour is acquired through learning and interacting with other members of our culture. Even those responses to our purely biological needs (i.e. eating, coughing, defecating) are frequently influenced by our cultures. Think of yourself and the culture you identify with.

(Continued)

(Continued)

Take time to reflect on how your culture governs the way in which you view the world and interact with others. How does your culture impact your values, beliefs and attitudes? To what extent are your cultural beliefs reflected in your nursing studies and the care that you participate in and receive?

Because this reflective exercise is of a highly personal nature, there is no outline answer at the end of the chapter. You might want to discuss your 'findings' with a trusted friend or colleague and make changes to your working practice according to your 'findings'.

Diversity among populations and people

Even within peoples and cultures, there is diversity. Diversity is any dimension that can be used to differentiate groups and people from one another. Diversity can be along the dimensions of race, ethnicity, gender, sexual orientation, socio-economic status, age, physical abilities, religious beliefs, political beliefs or other ideologies. It is anything that sets us aside from others. People from the same ethnic or racial group can also be 'diverse' in terms of socio-economic status, education, age, sexual orientation, individual experiences or disposition.

Discrimination, stigma and prejudice

Anything that marks us out as different opens us up to discrimination, stigma and prejudice. Discrimination means *treating a person unfairly because of who they are or because they possess certain characteristics* (EHRC, 2016). It is unlawful to behave in such a way to another person or group under the Equality Act 2010. Stigma refers to the negative qualities and perceptions that are attributed to people who are somehow different from others, whereas prejudice is a baseless and usually negative attitude towards members of a group. Common features of prejudice include negative feelings, stereotyped beliefs and a tendency to discriminate against members of the group. That is not to say that we are always conscious of our prejudices.

Conscious and unconscious bias

Bias is a prejudice in favour of or against one thing, person or group compared with another, usually in a way that is considered to be unfair.

Biases may be held by an individual, group or institution and can have negative or positive consequences. There are two types of biases:

1. conscious bias;
2. unconscious bias.

When we are consciously biased, we are doing it intentionally. We know we are being biased towards a particular person or group. Imagine you prefer working with men more than women, or you don't like working with young people or those with a different skin colour or culture. These are all dangerous prejudices. Most people now understand that there is no place for this in the modern workplace. Laws and policies exist to prevent prejudice based on race, age, gender, gender identity, physical abilities, religion, sexual orientation and many other characteristics.

Unconscious biases are social stereotypes about certain groups of people that individuals form outside their own conscious awareness. Everyone holds unconscious beliefs about various social and identity groups, and these biases stem from one's tendency to organise social worlds by categorising.

It is important to note that biases, conscious or unconscious, are not limited to ethnicity and race. Though racial bias and discrimination are well documented, biases may exist towards any social group (age, gender, gender identity, physical abilities, religion, sexual orientation, weight and many other characteristics are subject to bias).

Unconscious bias is far more prevalent than conscious bias, and often incompatible with one's conscious values. Certain scenarios can activate unconscious attitudes and beliefs. For example, biases may be more prevalent when multitasking or working under time pressure.

Unconscious bias can occur when we need to make decisions and judgements quickly and we are not thinking about what it is we are doing. We are not always making conscious decisions that are well thought through, taking all factors into account. Our brains work quickly, so they access information that is known and familiar to us first. This information is based on our personal experiences, meaning there is a natural bias towards views and opinions that fit the world view with which we are most familiar and comfortable. By doing this unconsciously, there is no malicious intent; we are often unaware that we have done it, as well as its impact and implications.

Health equity

Many magnitudes of disparity, particularly in healthcare, exist in the UK. There has been a growing recognition as to the depth of the problem in recent years, particularly in racial and ethnic **minority groups**. These groups experience poorer health compared to that of the rest of the population for a number of reasons. Various factors, such as race or ethnicity, gender, age, disability and socio-economic status, contribute to an individual's capability to attain good health (WHO, 2014). Health disparities are health differences between groups of people. These differences may include how many people are screened for a disease, whether people get healthcare and how many people die from a disease or condition. Reducing health disparities and promoting health equity is a major goal of public health and the focus of many health promotion campaigns and interventions.

Various studies since the COVID-19 pandemic began have found that people from Black, Asian and Minority Ethnic (BAME) groups have experienced disproportionately high levels of mortality relative to their white counterparts (Razaq et al., 2020). Haque, Becares & Treloar (2020) highlighted how structural issues such as the likelihood of poverty within BAME groups, living in substandard accommodation and other risk factors such as overcrowding and multi-generational households were all contributing factors towards the spread and poor containment of COVID-19 within these groups, making social isolation difficult for some families. These and other reports all demonstrate the existing health inequalities between groups of people and the inequitable starting point for how people survive a pandemic. An additional difficulty is that BAME is not one homogenous group, and the impact, development and recovery are different for different ethnic populations.

A report by Public Health England (2020b) titled *Analysis of the Relationship Between Pre-existing Health Conditions, Ethnicity and COVID-19* found that among people with one or more pre-existing health conditions, there were more COVID-19 cases in every ethnic minority group (apart from Chinese) than would be expected if they had the same rate of COVID-19 diagnoses as all people with the conditions.

Furthermore, there are several research studies that suggest three in every four adults of Black ethnicity are overweight or obese. Black and Asian ethnic groups also have much higher rates of diabetes, with some reports showing that BAME populations experience three to five higher prevalence than those of White ethnicity.

According to Office for National Statistics, regarding Coronavirus and vaccine hesitancy in Great Britain on 9 August 2021, Black or Black British adults had the highest rates of vaccine hesitancy (21 per cent) compared with White adults (4 per cent). When Great Britain was taken as a whole, those of Black or Black British ethnicity, the unemployed and those living in deprived areas were generally the most hesitant towards vaccines in all English regions.

Hesitancy in coming forward and receiving the COVID-19 vaccination among BAME groups could have owed something to the racial abuse and reported hate crimes towards these people (particularly those from Asian communities).

Equity has been defined as *the absence of avoidable unfair or remediable differences among groups of people, whether those groups are defined socially, economically, demographically or geographically or by other means of stratification* (WHO, 2019). Achieving health equity means treating people the same regardless of their race or ethnicity, gender, sexual identity, age, disability, socio-economic status and geographical location, as well as avoiding discriminating between groups of people. It requires valuing diversity and tackling injustices where found in healthcare. Efforts to eliminate disparities and achieve health equity have focused primarily on disease or illnesses and on healthcare services. However, the absence of disease does not automatically equate to good health, and differences continue to be had accessing and using health services among different peoples. Evidence suggests that these differences are widening, and that people and communities are becoming more socially isolated (HM Government, 2018a).

Concept Summary: Race and Ethnic Disparities

Structural racism and marginalisation cannot be ignored and was present before the pandemic. Whether it is accessing healthcare or finding work, the way society is run can reinforce inequalities and promote racial stereotyping. In 2021 the Commission on Race and Ethnic Disparities issued its report on Race and Ethnic Disparities in the UK. The Commission asked important questions about the state of race relations and provided a thorough examination of why so many disparities across different groups of peoples persist. The Commission made four major recommendations, these being:

- to build trust between different communities and the institutions that serve them;
- to promote greater fairness to improve opportunities and outcomes for individuals and communities;
- to create agency so that individuals can take greater control of the decisions that impact their lives;
- to achieve genuine inclusivity to ensure that all groups feel a part of UK society.

These recommendations are to be actioned through the social structures of health, education, training and skills, justice and policing. Of the recommendations relating to health, it is proposed that the government establish an Office for Health Disparities (Recommendation 11) and increase programmes aimed at levelling up healthcare and health outcomes (Recommendation 11a).

For further information and access to the full report, access the following link:

**https://assets.publishing.service.gov.uk/government/uploads/system/uploads/attach
ment_data/file/974507/20210331_-_CRED_Report_-_FINAL_-_Web_Accessible.pdf**

The recommendations relating to health make for challenging reading and highlight that there is still much work to be done in building relationships and achieving equality of service.

Vulnerable groups

Access to healthcare is an important goal of the NHS, but there are concerns that some vulnerable groups in the population have poorer access than others. A vulnerable group of people is one that experiences a higher risk of poverty and social exclusion than the general population. Ethnic minorities, migrants, traveller and gypsy populations, disabled people, the homeless, those living with a mental illness, those struggling with substance abuse, isolated elderly people and children all often face difficulties that can lead to further social exclusion, such as low levels of education and unemployment or underemployment (Atkinson, 2000).

Focus on homelessness

While all vulnerable groups are worthy of attention, this chapter will focus on the issue of homelessness, a growing problem in the UK. It has been estimated that there are as many as 320,000 homeless people in the UK (Shelter, 2018). Shelter estimated that on any given night in England in 2021 there were over 274 000 people who were homeless, which is a rate of 1 in 206 people. This means that you are likely to encounter someone who is homeless as you go about your everyday life. Homelessness is a complex social and economic problem that continues to persist and grow. An increasing shortage of affordable rental housing and a simultaneous rise in poverty are two trends largely responsible for the growth of homelessness over the past 10–20 years.

Poor health is both an effect and a cause of homelessness. Homelessness is associated with various behavioural, social and environmental risks that expose individuals to many diseases. People experiencing homelessness usually have complex health problems. Homeless people experience exposure to extremes in temperatures, unsanitary living conditions, crowded shelters, poor nutrition and unsafe situations wherever they live.

Within the context of poverty and the lack of affordable housing, other additional major factors, such as lack of affordable healthcare, domestic violence, mental illness and additional disorders, can also contribute to homelessness.

People who are homeless experience extreme stress on a daily basis. Multiple stresses of living in shelters and on the streets, physical problems, lack of resources, psychological issues such as shame and stigma and feelings of hopelessness and despair often tax the homeless person's ability to cope.

The prevalence of substance abuse among homeless people is much higher than that among the general population. Substance abuse is both a leading cause and a consequence of the continuance of homelessness among individuals.

Case study: Telli

Telli Afrik, his wife and two young children are a family caught up in the homelessness crisis. They lost their home, despite working, because they could no longer afford to pay the rent on their London flat. They are now living in a single room in their sixth homeless hostel and have to eat sitting on the floor because they have no table. Telli has lost his job as a supermarket manager because he has had to attend so many appointments with different housing teams and is not sure where they are going to end up next. 'My family are at breaking point,' he says. Telli is depressed and is finding that his and his family's physical health is deteriorating.

The definition of homelessness means not having a home. You are homeless if you have nowhere to stay and are living on the streets, but you can be homeless even if you have a roof over your head. You count as homeless if you are staying with friends or family, staying in a hostel, night shelter or B&B, squatting (because you have no legal right to stay), at risk of violence or abuse in your own home, living in poor conditions that affect your health or living apart from your family because you don't have a place to live together (Shelter, 2018).

The Housing (Homeless Persons) Act 1977, Housing Act 1996 and Homeless Act 2002 placed statutory duties on local housing authorities to ensure that advice and assistance to households who are homeless, or threatened with homelessness, is available free of charge.

A 'main homelessness duty' is owed where the local housing authority is satisfied that the applicant is eligible for assistance, unintentionally homeless and falls within a specified priority need group. Such statutorily homeless households are referred to as 'acceptances'.

The 'priority need groups' include households with dependent children or a pregnant woman and people who are vulnerable in some way (e.g. mental illness, physical disability). In 2002, an order made under the Housing Act 1996 extended the priority need categories to include applicants:

- aged 16 or 17;
- aged 18 to 20 who were previously in care;
- vulnerable as a result of time spent in care, in custody, or in HM Forces;
- vulnerable as a result of having to flee their home because of violence or the threat of violence.

Where a main duty is owed, the authority must ensure that suitable accommodation is available for the applicant and his or her household. The duty continues until a settled housing solution becomes available for them or some other circumstance brings the duty to an end. Where households are found to be intentionally homeless or not in priority need, the authority must make an assessment of their housing needs and provide advice and assistance to help them find accommodation for themselves.

Because societies continue to change and evolve, there will always be those who are excluded and suffer as a consequence. We will now look at the general difficulties faced by vulnerable groups and those facing discrimination when accessing health services, and what this means for health promotion practice.

Accessing healthcare

The most commonly reported barriers/potential barriers that people from diverse and vulnerable groups face encompass difficulties registering with health services, especially for primary care. This barrier can originate from outside the health service (e.g. lacking the necessary documentation to fulfil legal conditions for using health services) or from within the health system (e.g. the application of arbitrary rules such as declining to register those with no fixed address). Lack of understanding of medical jargon is another commonly reported barrier in the literature, along with poor functional literacy, compounding the difficulty of accessing information. Consequences of these issues include not being able to read written medication instructions, appointments or health promotion information. Using information technology (such as making or checking in for appointments) has been reported to be challenging and to cause embarrassment for some people (Taber et al., 2015).

Health literacy barriers

A key barrier to accessing and using health services for many diverse communities is knowing how to access and navigate health systems and being able to access and understand health information. People from minority ethnic groups tend to be less aware of what services are available and how to access them. However, it is important to recognise that this varies across different communities. More attention needs to be paid to ensuring that information is available in different languages and formats. This highlights the need for an integrated approach that includes written information, telephone helplines, outreach services and media campaigns (Taber et al., 2015).

Cultural and language barriers

The lack of availability of good-quality interpreting and translating services can make some people from minority ethnic groups especially reliant on link workers, in the form of local volunteers and bilingual workers in voluntary organisations, in order to access services.

Another common issue that seems to cause problems between healthcare staff and some minority groups involves the number of family members accompanying or visiting relatives receiving healthcare.

Other issues include the importance of same-gender healthcare professionals, especially for gender-sensitive problems such as sexual and reproductive healthcare; understanding that some healthcare topics, such as mental health and substance misuse, may be considered taboo topics, and thus need to be handled with privacy and confidentiality; and sensitivities around end-of-life/palliative care and cancer. Using health services for sensitive health needs can also be associated with stigma and a sense of shame.

Attitudes of professionals towards certain groups

Professionals can also create barriers to service use, particularly if they have stereotyped assumptions about the preferences of people from minority ethnic groups and the availability of other sources of support from within the family (Age UK, 2014). **Stereotypes** can lead not only to faulty beliefs, but they can also result in both prejudice and discrimination.

Engaging with communities as part of health promotion

Good engagement with communities is described as being continuous, inclusive, well-informed, fit for purpose, transparent, influential, reciprocal and proportionate (Coulter, 2009). This means that health promotion should be offered to all, regardless of background. Effective user engagement requires a recognition and understanding of the power differentials between the healthcare provider and those who are vulnerable. Healthcare providers and persons seeking care bring their individual cultures and health beliefs and values to the healthcare experience. Understanding the cultural underpinning of care is a challenging task because of the complexity and interaction between the person seeking care and the healthcare provider's cultural beliefs. It also requires a sensitivity to the needs of those from differing origins. Multifaceted interventions at different levels, tailored to specific settings and target groups, seem likely to change behaviour, improve general health perception and self-efficacy and promote independent living.

Specialist roles

Developing a specialist role to work with community members has been highlighted as an important development in engaging with people from different cultures and countries. This includes, for example, the involvement of community members as links between healthcare and the community, facilitating relationships or providing health information to targeted groups of individuals.

Outreach

These strategies focus on outreach to communities (or taking care to the community), largely by a range of teams of healthcare practitioners. The importance of positive relationships between providers and communities is highlighted. Some reports, however, raised the idea that outreach services may reinforce disengagement from mainstream health services by providing an alternative means of care (McFadden et al., 2018).

Cultural competence

A number of initiatives are focused on cultural awareness training for staff. Cultural competence is becoming an integral part of delivering quality healthcare services to an increasingly diverse population that includes people from all over the world. Tackling health inequalities is about exploration of differences in a safe, positive and nurturing environment that embraces diversity and promotes respect. Cultural competence is not acquired quickly or casually; rather, it requires an intentional examination of one's thoughts and behaviours: *The first step toward becoming culturally competent is realizing that you probably aren't* (Tanner and Allen, 2007, page 254). Cultural awareness is a person's understanding of the difference between themselves and people from other countries or backgrounds, especially differences in attitudes and values. Activity 8.2 helps to promote cultural awareness by asking you a series of short questions.

Activity 8.2   Reflection

Answer the following questions and reflect on them:

1. What race/ethnicity do you most closely associate with?
2. What represents the race/ethnicity of your significant other?
3. What represents the race of your closest friend?
4. 'My neighbours on either side of my house are ...'
5. 'My doctor is ...'
6. 'My boss is ...'
7. 'My co-workers are predominantly ...'
8. 'The people in my social circle are predominantly ...'
9. 'During the course of a day, the patients that I mainly come into contact with are ...'
10. 'The people in my favourite TV show are predominantly ...'
11. 'The author of the last book I read was ...'
12. 'The person who I most admire or who has had the greatest impact on my life is ...'
13. 'In the last movie I saw, the people were predominantly ...'
14. How culturally diverse are you?

Because this reflective exercise is of a highly personal nature, there is no outline answer at the end of the chapter. You might want to discuss your 'findings' with a trusted friend or colleague and make changes to your working practice according to your 'findings'.

Lifestyle and behaviour are central to the acquisition and development of major chronic diseases. To influence lifestyle and behaviour, health promoters must take into account the values, attitudes, culture and life circumstances of the individual. If we are to achieve salutary changes in the health status of minority populations, health professionals and designers of health programmes must cope with the extraordinary diversity of populations. Cultural competence is a dynamic, ongoing developmental process that requires a long-term commitment and is achieved over time, *a set of congruent behaviours, attitudes and policies that ... enable a system, agency or group of professionals to work effectively in cross-cultural situations* (Cross et al., 1989, page 13). It refers to the ability to honour and respect the beliefs, languages, interpersonal styles and behaviours of individuals and families receiving services, as well as staff members who are providing such services.

Achieving cultural competence requires the participation of racially and ethnically diverse groups and underserved populations in the development and implementation of treatment approaches and training activities. Organisational commitment to supporting culturally responsive treatment services, including adequate allocation of resources, reinforces the importance of sustaining cultural competence in nurses and other clinical staff. An understanding of race, ethnicity and culture (including one's own) is necessary to appreciate the diversity of human dynamics and to treat clients effectively. Incorporating cultural competence into treatment improves therapeutic decision making and offers alternative ways to define and plan a treatment programme firmly directed towards progress and recovery.

Chapter summary

This chapter has looked at the health of diverse and vulnerable populations. This is a hugely complex and challenging area of practice. Nurses need to become culturally competent if they are going to be able to work with people from differing backgrounds. There is a need to safeguard against stigma and ensure a high level of care, as well as being prepared to act as an advocate for those at a disadvantage.

Further reading

Shelter, *Homelessness in England 2021: The Numbers Behind the Story*. Available at: https://england.shelter.org.uk/professional_resources/policy_and_research/policy_library/homelessness_in_england_2021

Useful websites

www.gov.uk/government/publications/inclusion-health-applying-all-our-health/inclusion-health-applying-all-our-health

This guide is part of Public Health England's 'All Our Health' programme, a resource that helps health and care professionals prevent ill health and promote wellbeing as part of their everyday practice.

www.kingsfund.org.uk/topics/health-inequalities

The King's Fund is a leading research and think tank on matters of health. This link sends you to their work on health inequalities and access to care for different groups in society.

Chapter 9 Health promotion and emergent technologies

Annexe A: Communication and relationship management skills

At the point of registration, the registered nurse will be able to safely demonstrate the following skills:

2.5   identify the need for and manage a range of alternative communication techniques.

Chapter aims

After reading this chapter, you will be able to:

- describe the use of emergent technologies in health promotion;
- have an understanding of how emergent technologies can be used to promote health;
- develop an awareness of the challenges facing the use of emergent technologies in promoting health and well-being.

Case study: Maria

Maria asked her family if they would get her a **Fitbit** for her birthday. A Fitbit is a wearable device, often worn around the wrist like a watch, that provides feedback about the wearer's amount and intensity of activity during the course of a day. Maria had decided that she needed 'to get fit' and that she would start to walk more. At 44 years old, Maria did not want to take up jogging, nor did she want to join a gym, and joked that she didn't 'look good in Lycra'; besides which, she was put off by the price of the gym membership.

Maria works as an administrative assistant for a local company and spends most of her working day sitting at a computer. Before taking up walking, Maria would take the car to work and spend most evenings sitting in front of the television with her husband, Colin. Since getting the Fitbit, Maria has set herself the target of walking 10,000 steps a day. This is roughly the equivalent of five miles a day. Maria was 'sensible' and built up to this target, initially doing between 3,000 and 4,000 steps a day to 'get her going' and build up her fitness levels.

According to the NHS (2019d), the average Briton walks between 3,000 and 4,000 steps a day. This is an average and many people will walk significantly more steps; likewise, there will be some that do not walk much at all. Walking is simple, free and one of the easiest ways to get more active, lose weight and become healthier. The key to success is to incorporate it into your daily routine. Examples include walking part of your journey to work, walking to

(Continued)

(Continued)

the shops, using the stairs instead of the lift, leaving the car behind for short journeys, walking the children to school, doing a regular walk with a friend and going for a stroll with family or friends after dinner.

Maria's husband has now started going out walking with her in the evening and he too says that he is benefiting from getting more exercise.

Introduction

A considerable number of people are now wearing fitness devices and using them to monitor their health and well-being as part of their daily exercise routine. Wearable fitness devices can act as a motivator for people to take up more exercise as part of their daily routine, as in the case of Maria and Colin above (Coughlin and Stewart, 2016). These devices offer numerous features that promote greater engagement among users and make being physically active more fun (Patel et al., 2015). Such incentives include options for personal goal setting, rewards for achieving milestones and the ability to connect, compete and interact with peers and give or receive social support through **mobile application interfaces**, as well as the capacity to track activity and individual performance over time through user-friendly graphs (Lyons et al., 2014). Encouraging physical activity and making it accessible and feasible to individuals and groups of people is an important public health objective.

This chapter discusses the use of technology-enabled care (TEC) by nurses and other healthcare professionals. TEC involves the convergence of health and information technologies, digital media and mobile devices in support of health and well-being. It seeks to illustrate the benefits to be had from such technologies and why it is important that nurses should engage with them as part of health promotion practice. As part of this, the chapter will explore the key barriers and challenges to using such technologies as part of clinical practice. It will also look at what it means to live a healthy life in a digital age. The chapter ends with a look at some of the overriding issues when accessing and using information, including issues of security, confidentiality and information governance, which continue to present challenges when introducing new technologies into the workplace.

TEC-enabled health promotion

If there is one thing that has brought the globe together then it is surely the rise of technologies, particularly mobile technologies in support of daily living. Opportunities for using mobile technology have increased one hundredfold over the last ten years and particularly during COVID-19. The population of smartphone and tablet users has grown, supported by a proliferation of health apps. Most notable are the availability of healthcare biosensing wearables, such as blood pressure sensors, and patient and provider access to real-time healthcare data and information. Additionally, smartphones and smart technology are incorporating a growing range of sensors which monitor not only changes in physiology, but mood and emotional well-being.

Mobile technology can empower patients and carers by giving them more control over their health and well-being and making them less dependent on care services. Patients can use digital technology to research information online, share experiences and identify support and treatment options, as well as prompting higher levels of functioning and independence. Other aspects of the growing use of TEC are remote monitoring or changes to health status of patients (e.g. home telehealth) and the use of digital messages to remind or alert patients to adhere to their long-term course of treatment or therapy (particularly in Mental Health Services).

From its early inception, healthcare digital technologies were seen as having the potential for improving the delivery of quality healthcare by providing up-to-the-minute, real-time information about a patient's condition necessary for decision making. Initially, the incorporation of new technologies was fundamentally used for administrative tasks involving data storage and statistics. Later, however, technologies gradually began to be used to save personal records and clinical summaries, giving healthcare practitioners access to data on individuals and diagnostic, preventative and health maintenance information that they could even share with colleagues.

There is no doubt that the use of digital technology and the use of TEC have the power to transform health and social care and improve quality, efficiency and the patient experience, as well as supporting more integrated care and improving the health of a population (Maguire et al., 2018). Its use in providing access to information and education is an important driver of patient engagement and has helped to bridge the gap between hospitals and the community. The potential use of TECs continues to grow with the development of high-speed and wireless connections, decreasing cost and the technology boom in smart technology whereby different technologies and devices can 'talk to each other'. This has allowed for the creation of care environments that not only monitor the safety and well-being of individuals, but respond to the changing needs of the person in 'real-time' (e.g. creating safe environments for people living with dementia) (Wenzel and Evans, 2019).

TEC is an umbrella term for telecare, telehealth, telemedicine, mHealth, digital health and eHealth. TEC covers everything from wearable devices to ingestible sensors, from mobile phone apps to artificial intelligence, from robotic carers to electronic records and everything in between. These new forms of delivery produce new contents of care, such as 'blended' care, where conventional healthcare is combined with online interventions. These emergent technologies challenge not only the way that clinicians talk to each other and share information, but also the way that care is organised and delivered. As the use and development of TEC grows, so too does the potential to move hands-on care and treatments in primary care clinics and hospitals to home care via the use of digital communication such as e-visits, e-prescriptions and remote monitoring as witnessed during the COVID-19 pandemic when people went into lockdown. Many such technologies are now explicitly designed for medical and health purposes (Wahl et al., 2019). Mobile digital devices and the applications ('apps'), websites and platforms to which they connect offer not only ready access to medical and health information on the internet, but also new ways of monitoring, measuring and visualising the human body, as well as sharing personal information and experiences with others.

While the reported benefits of TECs are well documented (e.g. improved information management, access to health services, quality improvement, cost containment), their effects have yet to be fully realised (Cherrill and Linsley, 2017). Some of this is down to healthcare not keeping pace with changes in technology, some of this is staff not wanting to change their practice and some of this is down to cost. During the coming decade, the speed, scope and scale of adoption of health TEC will only increase (Menefee et al., 2016). Think about how technology shapes your day-to-day clinical practice by completing Activity 9.1.

Activity 9.1   Reflection

Make a list of all the digital devices and electronic information and communication systems that you come into contact with and use as part of clinical practice over the course of a shift. To what extent do they aid and support clinical practice? What are the benefits of using them? Could better use be made of them? Are there difficulties with using them?

Because this is a reflective exercise, there is no outline answer at the end of the chapter. The hope is that it has raised your awareness of how such technologies impact on your daily clinical practice.

It is important to acknowledge at this point the limitations imposed by digital poverty and digital literacy. Technology and digital health have advanced at such a rapid rate that many of us take for granted the ease and convenience that it brings, forgetting that it comes at a cost. Not everyone can afford the latest technology and software. Likewise, there are many adults who lack essential digital skills for life and work. The impact of this means tasks such as accessing healthcare and support, applying for a job or social housing to managing finances are simply not an option.

Health TEC Promotion

Health TEC Promotion, as outlined in further detail below, includes a range of digital devices and technologies, tools and platforms that support health-promoting practices and activities. Some of these practices are voluntarily undertaken by people who are interested in improving their health and fitness, but many others are employed for the broader purposes of organisations and agencies, both corporate and governmental (WHO, 2016).

Mobile applications (mHealth) and internet of things (IoT)

mHealth is a general term for the practice of medicine and care delivery that is supported by the use of mobile phones and other wireless technology (DHI, 2019). With increased access to mobile technology, such as tablets (e.g. iPad), mHealth offers the potential to promote better health and help people to achieve a healthier lifestyle. With mHealth, there are so many possible applications, including, but not limited to, education, diagnostic support, helplines and remote monitoring and data collection. Improvements in mobile phone signals and access to broadband have increased the range of devices that can be used, especially in rural areas.

The use of mobile applications and devices is further enhanced when connected to the internet of things. The internet of things describes any devices that are embedded with sensors, software and other technologies for the purpose of connecting and exchanging data with other devices and systems over the internet, including big data analytics. Big data analytics being the examination of large data to uncover patterns, correlations, trends and other insights in population health. Knowledge about disease trends and other threats to community health can improve programme planning, decision making, care delivery and support for populations. Thus, mHealth ranges from the simple, single-use applications to complex monitoring and predictive modelling activities (see Table 9.1).

Domain	Example
1 Single use mHealth. Mobile devices and items often for personal use only.	For example, Smartphone apps to monitor and record personal health data, which the person may or may not share with others.
2 Social mHealth devices and technology that promote social support and encouragement.	For example, support and competition-based apps where personal data is shared with likeminded others as part of social networks with the aim to encourage and support the individual to achieve certain health targets.
3 Integrated mHealth. Formal use of apps and devices as part of a healthcare system or service.	For example, systematised use of patient and population electronically stored health information shared by healthcare providers across different settings and disciplines e.g. electronic health records.
4 Complex mHealth to support population health decision making.	For example, the use of population health data gathered from a number of mobile devices and subjected to complex data analysis with the aim of improving public health. We saw this through the tracking of COVID-19 cases and uptake of vaccination programmes across different age groups in terms of effectiveness and protection against the COVID-19 virus.

Table 9.1 mHealth: from simple to complex (adapted from Four Dimensions of Effective mHealth, Deloitte US Center for Health Solutions (2014))

Telehealth and telephony

Telehealth involves the use of telecommunications and virtual technology to deliver healthcare and support outside of the traditional healthcare facilities. Telehealth examples include virtual healthcare, where patients such as the chronically ill or elderly may receive guidance in certain procedures while remaining at home (EC, 2018). Telephony is any technology associated with interactive communication between two or more physically distant parties via electronic transmission (e.g. the telephone). Telehealth is the use of such technology in support of healthcare activities, including text messaging, video calling, video conferencing and increasingly **chatbots**. Telehealth has come to the fore during COVID-19, having allowed health professionals to support patients when the population was in lockdown.

SMART Technology

As we have already seen, emerging wearable devices and smartphone applications afford opportunities for promoting physical activity, as well as the monitoring and management of certain conditions, and they are now being actively incorporated into weight reduction programmes, exercise programmes and the monitoring of such things as anxiety levels in people with a mental health problem. Wearable devices and the smartphone applications connected with these devices are increasing in popularity, availability and affordability and are now in common use for a number of people (Naylor et al., 2016).

Case study: Grace

Grace is a 76-year-old woman who suffers from high blood pressure. Grace is also forgetful and will sometimes forget to take her blood pressure tablets. This results in her going dizzy and having to sit down and take a rest, as well as at times having to seek the support and help of others. Grace has now set the alarm on her mobile phone to remind her when to take her medication. This simple step means that she now remembers to take her medication as prescribed and is more confident in going out of the house, something that she had been avoiding doing for 'fear of collapsing'. A lot of health promotion is about making small changes.

As with Grace, many people are using mainstream devices such as smartphones to help them in their daily lives. This might be as simple as setting a daily reminder to have something to eat and drink, to take medication or to be notified of an upcoming medical appointment.

Personal self-tracking and monitoring devices

The development of wireless mobile devices and associated software that can monitor and measure many aspects of body functions and activities, as well as geolocation details, has provided people with the opportunity to engage in self-tracking (Lupton, 2014). Body functions, sensations and indicators such as blood glucose (see case study below), body weight and body mass index, physical activity, energy expended, mood, body temperature, breathing rate, blood chemistry readings and even brain activity can now all be monitored using portable, wearable and internal sensors that have been embedded in wristbands or headbands, woven into clothing, laminated on to ultrathin skin interfaces or inserted into ingestible tablets that can monitor the body from within. These technologies produce detailed data that may be readily communicated to others via social media platforms or to medical or public health professionals monitoring people's biometrics and health-related habits (see case study below). With rapid advances in technology, functionality and size, wearables offer great potential for personalised treatment and care.

Case study: Sally

Sally is 21 years old. She leads a full and active life and really enjoys sports. Sally is type 2 diabetic and wears a continuous glucose monitor which she had fitted in consultation with her diabetic nurse. A continuous glucose monitor is a small device that you wear just under your skin. It measures your glucose (sugar) levels continuously throughout the day and night, letting you see trends in your levels, and alerts you to highs and lows. It sends this information to a display device using Bluetooth.

The information collected about Sally's blood sugar levels can be accessed instantly and shared with her healthcare team so that they can review and adjust her treatment appropriately. It also means that the information can be shared easily during virtual appointments with her healthcare team.

Assistive technology

It is important to remember that health promotion is not just about helping to treat people, but also helping people to achieve their optimum health and maintain good health, as well as promoting independent living. Assistive technology can be any piece of kit that helps you get on with your daily life and promotes independent living. This normally means electronic technology, gadgets or sensors that are designed to prompt you or raise alarm if something goes wrong. Sensor-based technologies are expanding in domestic and urban environments.

'Smart' objects embedded with sensors can be installed in people's homes to monitor their physical activity. This is becoming a feature of home-based care for elderly people (Majumder et al., 2017). A sensor network is a network of spatially distributed autonomous devices, such as electronic cameras using sensors to co-operatively monitor physical or environmental conditions. Homes can also be designed to monitor their inhabitants' use of energy, as well as linking the sleep data collected by wearable devices of their inhabitants to engineer energy use to coincide with going to bed and waking up. Smart environments have the potential to allow users to engage and interact seamlessly with their immediate surroundings. This has been made possible by the introduction of intelligent technologies coupled with software-based services.

'Smart' homes can benefit from artificial intelligence (AI), which can gather and analyse information regarding the occupant's activities and health status, as well as identifying and reporting any anomalies (Majumder et al., 2017). The AI system includes a database that stores residents' behavioural and physiological patterns and medical histories. In case of a medical emergency, this system can raise an alarm and share medical profiles with the concerned authority over a secure channel, thus allowing the residents to have immediate and appropriate medical attention.

Case study: John

John is a 62-year-old man who is recovering from having suffered a left-sided stroke. He lives with his wife, Susan, in their two-bedroom bungalow and generally manages around the house. John is making a good recovery and is mobilising and attending to his own physical needs.

Susan still works and is worried about John when she is not with him. John's main problem is that he is forgetful at times. Every now and then, John will leave the house and walk up the road to the shops by himself. Motion and heat sensors have been attached to the front door in case John forgets to close it when he goes out. These send an alert to Susan's mobile phone; she then rings John to see if he is all right. If there is no response from John, Susan can ring their daughter, Jane, who lives nearby, to pop round and see if her dad is OK, as well as closing the door and securing the house if need be.

Treatment and therapies online

There are now a number of downloadable mental health software applications ('apps') for use with mobile phones and other portable devices covering a wide range of treatment interventions and assessment tools (Cotton et al., 2014). Mobile phone applications such as Skype have opened new avenues and possibilities in telehealth and telemedicine, whereby engagement with the patient is done over distance, cutting down on the travelling times and costs for patients, their families and health service personnel, meaning that the nurse and other members of the multidisciplinary team can 'see' more patients in a day.

There are apps to aid diagnosis and assessment, monitor treatment progress and evaluate the effectiveness of interventions. There are lifestyle apps to give advice on healthy living and apps to help people quit smoking and lose weight. There are now complete courses of cognitive behavioural therapies available online, which people can access and pay for from the comfort of their own home. However, these do require the individual to have motivation and sustain engagement if they are to work (Bennett et al., 2017).

Perhaps the biggest strength of such devices and technology is the breaking down of social isolation. Australia has had a large degree of success combatting social isolation in the elderly population by issuing iPads to those of pensionable age who live away from their relatives (Feist et al., 2012).

Case study: Michelle

Michelle is a 15-year-old girl who suffers from mood swings. When depressed, emotionally distressed or upset, Michelle engages in self-injurious behaviour. Michelle began cutting herself at age 13. Initially she cut herself on her forearms, but then switched to her upper thighs to conceal the injuries. Michelle's primary reason for engaging in self-injury was to release built-up emotional pressure. Episodes typically occurred after an emotional conflict with her parents or a perceived rejection by a peer.

Adolescence is a period notable for substantial emotional and behavioural challenges that correspond with important brain developmental changes. When adolescents experience strong negative emotions, they experiment with a range of coping behaviours, some of which may be maladaptive, such as substance use, disordered eating patterns and nonsuicidal self-injury. Michelle is being supported by the community mental health team and is making good progression.

Michelle monitors her mood by the use of a 'mood diary' and uses an app as a reminder of what to do to when thinking of cutting herself. This includes a series of exercises that encourage Michelle to explore and challenge her thoughts and adopt more positive ways of coping with her fluctuations in mood.

She has utilised a variety of techniques and found that self-soothing strategies are particularly effective for regulating her emotions. Her interpersonal relationships have matured, with an improvement in perspective-taking and an accompanying decrease in interpersonal sensitivity and hostility. At extreme times Michelle can text and chat to the mental health team for support.

Social media

Social media platforms such as Twitter, Facebook, YouTube and Instagram have been developed, allowing for the creation of content and the sharing of personal data by users. They have challenged how we think about relationships and how we communicate with one another, and they have made the world a much smaller place.

Furthermore, social media play an increasingly important part in the way that the public search for, understand and use health information, significantly influencing their health decisions and actions. Healthcare organisations are increasingly using social media for communication and information sharing with their patients and the wider community.

Concept summary: social media

Perhaps the greatest advancements in health promotion have come about at the expansion and use of social media. Social media are the process of people using online tools and platforms to share content and information through conversation and communication. Social media:

- allow a wide variety of content formats (e.g. text, photos, video);
- are device-independent (e.g. computers, tablets, mobile phones/smartphones);
- facilitate speed and breadth of information dissemination;
- provide one-to-one, one-to-many and many-to-many communication;
- permit synchronous (existing or occurring at the same time) and asynchronous (not existing or occurring at the same time) communication;
- allow different levels of engagement.

(Bajwa, 2014)

While the use of social media technology creates possible opportunities for patient–nurse exchanges, through texting, e-mail or other exchange media formats, it raises new concerns regarding documentation and confidentiality.

Health information

Ideas about health and behaviours are shaped by the communication, information and technology that people interact with every day. Health communication and health information technology are central to healthcare, public health and the way our society views health (Thimbleby, 2013). The networking capability of online platforms brings together people with interests in health and care within countries and across borders to support each other, share learning and even provide a platform for tracking their health data or helping them manage their conditions. There is now a number of platforms that house an array of information and support the interests of a number of self-help groups.

Some social media platforms have been developed for the express purpose of sharing and crowdsourcing health-related information for the collective good. Platforms such as HealthMap and Sickweather encourage users to contribute information about their own or others' illnesses to generate geolocation data that can warn people when there is an infectious disease outbreak in their area. Platforms such as PatientsLikeMe, for people with health conditions, encourage the sharing of condition-specific symptoms and treatments by patients with one another. The role of the nurse is to help the patient evaluate these sites and make judgements based on good evidence. Activity 9.2 looks at an evaluation framework when judging the quality of a site.

Activity 9.2 Critical thinking

There is so much information available on the internet on every topic imaginable. But how do you know if it is any good? There are seven distinct aspects of information quality to consider when accessing information on the internet: audience, presentation, relevance, objectivity, method, provenance and timeliness (or for short, A PROMPT). Let us look at the seven aspects, one by one.

Audience

- Who is the website's intended audience? Academics? The general public? Schoolchildren?
- Does it appropriately address the target audience?
- Is it relevant for your assignment or research?

Presentation

By presentation, we mean the way in which the information is communicated. Ask yourself:

- Is the language clear and easy to understand?
- Is the information clear and easy to understand?
- If there are graphics or photos, do they help to communicate the information?
- If there is audio or video, is it clear?
- What about the use of animation? Is it helpful or distracting?

Relevance

Relevance is an important factor to consider when you are evaluating information. It is not so much a property of information itself, but of the relationship it has with your question or your 'information need'.

Objectivity

One of the characteristics of 'good information' is that it should be balanced and present both sides of an argument or issue. This way, the reader is left to weigh up the evidence and make a decision. In reality, we recognise that no information is truly objective.

(Continued)

(Continued)

This means that the onus is on you, the reader, to develop a critical awareness of the positions represented in what you read, as well as taking account of this when you interpret the information. In some cases, authors may be explicitly expressing a particular viewpoint; this is perfectly valid, as long as they are explicit about the perspective they represent. Hidden bias, whether or not it is deliberate, can be misleading. This could be particularly important in a subject area where there is controversy.

Method

Method is about the way in which a piece of information is produced. This is quite a complex area as different types of information are produced in different ways. These are some suggestions to look out for:

- *Opinions:* A lot of information is based on the opinion of individuals. They may or may not be experts in their field (see 'P' for provenance), but the key message is to be clear that it is just an opinion and must be valued as such.
- *Research:* You do not have to be an expert on research methods to ask some basic questions about research information. You need to develop a critical approach to reports for research, particularly when they are summarised by the popular media.

Provenance

The provenance of a piece of information (i.e. who produced it, where it came from) may provide another useful clue to its reliability. It represents the 'credentials' of a piece of information that support its status and value. It is therefore very important to be able to identify the author, sponsoring body or source of your information.

Now pick a topic of interest to you and look for a site promoting this topic on the internet. Having found a site, access the information it provides using the 'A PROMPT' framework above. Would you recommend the site to one of your patients? If so, why? If not, why not?

Timeliness

The date when information was produced or published can be an important aspect of quality. Is it clear when the information was produced? Does the date of the information meet your requirements? Is it out of date?

Because this activity is of personal interest, there is no outline answer at the end of the chapter.

Barriers to using Information and Communication Technologies (ICTs) in clinical practice

Despite the increasing demand on health to make use of advances in ICTs, there remains a number of barriers to their implementation. Key barriers to successful digital change include the constraints that care organisations face in their workforce, tight budgets, organisations' attitudes towards risk and the relationships that exist between care providers and key stakeholders (Maguire et al., 2018). ICTs come with a cost. Financial and business barriers remain, particularly when accessing and using new technologies. Training staff in the use of new technologies is another big barrier. Issues with training are invariably underestimated and commonplace in the implementation of ICTs. Tied to this are technical and professional barriers. Often there is a need to upskill nurses in the use of ICTs. Structural barriers, both physical and technological, remain (e.g. who gets what information, in what format, for what purposes). Perhaps the biggest barrier is the staff themselves. From the perspective of the nurse, the most frequently mentioned barrier is, 'I haven't got time for this'. Furthermore, nurses fear that it will depersonalise healthcare, and more specifically will interfere with their rapport with their patients. Lastly, the perceived threat to patient privacy and confidentiality remains a prominent concern.

Concept summary: The 10Es in e-health

While the 'e' in e-health stands for electronic, it has also been suggested by Eysenbach (2001), a leading medical writer on e-health, that it might also stand for other qualities which characterise what e-health is all about (or what it *should* be), a bit like the **6Cs** for nursing. These 10Es are useful for thinking about the use of ICTs in clinical practice:

1. *Efficiency*: One of the promises of e-health is to increase efficiency in healthcare, thereby decreasing costs. One possible way of decreasing costs would be by avoiding duplicative or unnecessary diagnostic or therapeutic interventions through enhanced communication possibilities between healthcare establishments, as well as through patient involvement.
2. *Enhancing quality of care*: Increasing efficiency involves not only reducing costs, but at the same time improving quality. E-health may enhance the quality of healthcare (e.g. allowing comparisons between different providers, involving consumers as additional power for quality assurance, directing patient streams to the best quality providers).
3. *Evidence-based*: E-health interventions should be evidence-based in the sense that their effectiveness and efficiency should not be assumed but proven by rigorous scientific evaluation.
4. *Empowerment of consumers and patients*: By making the knowledge bases of medicine and personal electronic records accessible to consumers over the internet, e-health opens new avenues for patient-centred medicine and enables evidence-based patient choice.
5. *Encouragement* of a new relationship between the patient and health professional, towards a true partnership, where decisions are made in a shared manner.
6. *Education* of physicians and other healthcare professionals through online sources (e.g. continuing professional development) and consumers (e.g. health education, tailored preventative information for consumers).

(Continued)

(Continued)

7. *Enabling* information exchange and communication in a standardised way between healthcare establishments.

8. *Extending the scope of healthcare beyond its conventional boundaries:* This is meant in both a geographical and conceptual sense. E-health enables consumers to easily obtain health services online from global providers. These services can range from simple advice to more complex interventions or products such as pharmaceuticals.

9. *Ethics:* E-health involves new forms of patient–clinician interaction and poses new challenges and threats to ethical issues, such as online professional practice, informed consent and privacy and equity issues.

10. *Equity:* To make healthcare more equitable is one of the promises of e-health, but at the same time there is a considerable threat that e-health may deepen the gap between the 'haves' and 'have-nots'. People who do not have money, skills and access to computers and networks cannot use computers effectively. As a result, these patient populations, who would actually benefit the most from health information, are those who are the least likely to benefit from advances in information technology, unless political measures ensure equitable access for all.

Going forward

There is no doubt that TEC has moved on since their inception and we are living in a technologically advanced age. If such technological systems are to meet the needs of the nurse in clinical practice, then the nurse needs to rethink how they use ICTs in meeting people's demands for health promotion. The nurse's role becomes one of creating opportunities for the use of existing technology in support of clinical practice (Jordan et al., 2018). Nurses should be skilled enough in the use of information and communication technologies to manage their information requirements in a way that sustains their specific area of practice for the betterment of their patients.

The real benefit to using technological advances in support of health promotion lies in their ability to empower the patient to take responsibility for their own health. Technological applications are very much part of people's lives, and it is important that the nurse recognises this. The increasing availability and advances in applications offer the opportunity to develop and adjust technological solutions to all aspects of healthcare, not just health promotion. The widespread use of the internet and mobile phones is currently challenging the way patients are educated, supported and followed up and it is almost an expectation of the public that technology will feature in their care and treatment in some way.

As the popularity of technology increases, patients are likely to expect to use them both in their care and as a means of communicating with healthcare professionals. Using such systems has implications for confidentiality; however, these are not unsurmountable. It should also be remembered that no system is completely foolproof. Data breaches have been known to occur when using paper systems.

Chapter summary

This chapter has raised your awareness of the use of TEC in health promotion and health service delivery. It has looked at the complexities of introducing such technologies into the workplace, as well as the need of the nurse to be up to date with advances in technology and to challenge how they use such technology in the care and support of the people they come into contact with. We have seen how the use of TEC can have a positive effect on patient engagement and how such technologies have changed the way that we think about health promotion. Going forward, there is a real need for nurses not only to keep up to date with such technologies, but to think creatively about how they use them when promoting the health of others.

Useful websites

www.cieh.org/ehn/

Environmental Health News is provided by the Chartered Institute of Environmental Health, and covers such issues as environmental protection, housing and community and public health and protection, and is of interest to both the health professional and the general public.

www.dh.gov.uk/en/index.htm

The Department of Health website, which has a dedicated public health banner filled with resources.

https://digital.nhs.uk/about-nhs-digital/our-work/digital-inclusion/what-digital-inclusion-is?key=

For more information on digital inclusion, digital poverty and digital literacy then follow access the NHS Digital works for digital inclusion.

www.frontiersin.org/journals/digital-health

While there is no one paper that we would suggest you read, you might like to access *Frontiers in Digital Health*, a multidisciplinary open-access journal that publishes rigorously peer-reviewed research in its field:

www.healthtechdigital.com/technology/

The site covers all the exciting topics on digital health in the UK and is worth spending time exploring. It is dedicated to UK healthcare technology, digital health and NHS technology, news and information.

www.nhs.uk/Pages/HomePage.aspx

NHS Choices (we particularly recommend the 'Live Well' section of the site as it is easy to navigate and is regularly updated).

www.patient.co.uk/showdoc/16

This site provides health and well-being information on a number of common conditions. Aimed at patients, it uses clear, easy-to-understand language. Very easy to access and navigate.

Chapter 10 Evaluating health promotion

NMC Future Nurse: Standards of Proficiency for Registered Nurses

This chapter will address the following platforms and proficiencies:

Platform 4: Providing and evaluating care

At the point of registration, the registered nurse will be able to:

4.3 demonstrate the knowledge, communication and relationship management skills required to provide people, families and carers with accurate information that meets their needs before, during and after a range of interventions.

Platform 7: Co-ordinating care

At the point of registration, the registered nurse will be able to:

7.4 identify the implications of current health policy and future policy changes for nursing and other professions and understand the impact of policy changes on the delivery and co-ordination of care.

Chapter aims

After reading this chapter, you will be able to:

- define what is meant by evaluation;
- describe the fundamental concepts and skills needed to undertake an evaluation of practice;
- identify approaches to conducting an evaluation.

Community nurse Sharon Bradford and community physiotherapist Ben Hale have been working with Hilda, an 82-year-old lady, and her husband, Tom, to 'get Hilda walking again'. Tom fears that Hilda has been isolating herself in the house following a recent hip replacement operation and that this is having an impact on her mood and social well-being. Hilda was an active person prior to her hip replacement but is now restricting herself to the house as she is fearful of going outside, falling over and 'needing another operation'.

Working in a person-centred way, the nurse supports and respects the wishes of the individual while promoting a range of interventions to promote health and well-being. Hilda is encouraged to mobilise with the aim of returning to a level of functioning whereby she is independent of Tom and can walk unaided and socialise as she wishes. But how does the nurse, and more importantly Hilda in this scenario, know that these interventions are having an effect and are achieving what they are supposed to be achieving? In other words, how do you, as a nurse, go about judging the effectiveness of the care that you give?

Introduction

The importance of promoting health and keeping healthy has never been more apparent. COVID-19 has had a profound effect on the way we view and live our lives, and it is said that its legacy will be with us for many years to come. These include changes in needs, habits and behaviours – whether it is less physical activity or shifting levels of mental well-being tied to uncertainties, the problems of working from home, or the social isolation and difficulties with missing friends and families. If nothing else, the COVID-19 pandemic has taught us the importance of health promotion and disease prevention and why it is important to stay healthy and keep disease at bay.

COVID-19 brought a number of challenges and changed our way of thinking, with regards to our health and well-being. Many health promotion initiatives and activities were introduced during the pandemic, often in quick succession; for example, the taking to wearing of face masks, social distancing, changes to vaccination rollout and new initiatives aimed at improving people's mental health.

There are many questions we can ask about the care and treatment that we give and promote. For any disease, there are usually several possible treatment options; for any service, there are many ways in which it may be organised; and for any health promotion intervention, there are a range of activities and approaches that might be adopted and actioned. How, then, are decisions to be taken and choices made between alternative treatments, different approaches and organisational arrangements? How do we know that the care and support we give is effective, timely, efficient and meets the needs of the individual?

Evaluating and assessing the impact of health promotion interventions allows us to learn and improve services and can inform future policy. Evaluation is recognised as a research approach in its own right and is used extensively in both health and social care, as well as in education, to maintain and improve the quality of programmes and activity (Linsley & Kane, 2022). While evaluation comes in many shapes and sizes, and is undertaken for a number of differing reasons, its main purpose is to help us develop a deeper understanding of the care that we provide, as well as helping to drive clinical practice forward.

The following chapter does not seek to take you step by step through the evaluation process; that would require more words than are available here. Instead, it is designed to get you thinking about the topic under investigation, as well as how you might go about approaching an evaluation in clinical practice as part of a health promotion intervention. It starts by exploring what we mean by evaluation and why we might choose to undertake an evaluation of a health promotion intervention. The main body of the chapter looks at the role of the nurse in supporting evaluation initiatives and the process of conducting them, as well as looking at the types of evaluation available to clinical practice. The chapter ends with a summary of the key points and considerations for future practice.

Defining evaluation

Evaluation has been defined in different ways for different purposes. A common definition, popular in the literature, defines evaluation as *the process of determining merit, worth or significance; an evaluation is a product of that process* (Scriven, 1991, page 53).

This definition suggests that if you evaluate something or someone, you consider them in order to make a judgement about them (e.g. how good or bad they are). Without proper safeguards, this process could be influenced by personal feelings, tastes or opinions in the form of **personal bias**. In order to safeguard against bias, evaluation should be conducted following the same rules as a research study and be conducted in a systematic way. We see support for this in the World Health Organization's definition of evaluation, in which they defined evaluation as *the systematic examination and assessment of the features of an initiative and its effects, in order to produce information that can be used by those who have an interest in its improvement or effectiveness* (WHO, 1998, page 3).

With an increasing drive for quality, the definition of healthcare evaluation has been expanded to include elements of service improvement and cost-effectiveness. Evaluation of any service or care should be about *checking that you are doing things right* and *checking that you are doing the right thing*, at the 'right cost' (NHS Institute for Innovation and Improvement, 2005, page 4).

An assumption underpinning this chapter is that evaluation is an analytical process and one that is intrinsic to good care. For the purposes of this book, the authors define evaluation as *the process of critically reviewing the efficiency (did we do the right thing?) and effectiveness of an activity (did we do it in the best possible way?) in a manner that was timely and met the needs of the person or service (including cost).*

By following a process, evaluation can be used to help in the design of services, to access how well the services are working and to find out whether services are effective in what they do. Conducting a good evaluation can help us to understand the impact of an activity, whether things need to be changed during delivery, adapted for next time or stopped altogether. It can also help to move practice forward and, if communicated in the right way, help steer the development of new policies and new ways of working (King's Fund, 2018b). It also has an important part to play in promoting **evidence-based practice**. Evaluation that is done inadequately, or not done at all, can render an intervention at best a wasted effort, with improvements only realised at a local level (Health Foundation, 2015, page 5). An evaluation of clinical practice might be undertaken for several reasons; the following activity gets you to consider some of these.

Activity 10.1   Critical thinking

There are a number of reasons why you might wish to conduct an evaluation as part of your work. Can you think of some? Make a list of why you might want to undertake an evaluation of your own clinical practice.

Compare your list with the outline answer at the end of the chapter.

What the activity demonstrates is that evaluation is part of everyday clinical practice. Often an evaluation of a service or intervention is undertaken because we are told to do so or because we have a personal interest in the results and think that it is a good idea. Whatever your reasons, you need to be clear on what you are being asked to evaluate and why. All evaluation should be purposeful and serve the interests of others as well as yourself. It should not be conducted in a way that can only produce the answer you want, but ideally should inform your own and others' clinical practice.

Evaluation as part of the nursing process

The importance of evaluation is highlighted in the nursing process. The nursing process has been used for a number of years to guide the actions of nurses in clinical practice when planning and implementing care. It remains a foundation on which nursing practice is based and is taught to nursing students the world over (Miskir and Emishaw, 2018). The approach can be remembered by the use of the acronym APIE (assess, plan, implement and evaluate).

Concept Summary: AIPE

Table 10.1 is an example of a care plan based on a health education approach.

Assess	• Assess the person's individual perceptions of their health problems.
	• Assess the person's learning needs.
	• Assess cultural influences on health teaching.
	• Assess the person's confidence in their ability to perform the desired behaviour / change (e.g. change of diet).
Plan	• Clearly define the specific behaviour to be addressed / changed.
	• Assist the person in developing a time frame for implementation of specific behaviour.
	• Identify possible barriers to change (e.g. lack of motivation, interpersonal support, skills, knowledge or resources).
	• Plan for lapses and relapses.
Implement	• Provide specific instruction on topics or behaviours (e.g. smoking cessation, weight loss, promoting good hygiene).
	• Use a variety of teaching methods to match the person's preferred learning style.
	• Inform the person of community resources and self-help groups as appropriate.
	• Encourage the participation of family or significant others as appropriate.
Evaluate	• How successful was the person in implementing the desired behaviour / change?
	This will often take the form of measurable behaviours and self-reporting measures e.g. the person lost a given weight, attended and participated in a twice-weekly exercise class over a set period of time and this was recorded in their health diary.

Table 10.1 A care plan based on a health education approach

Reassessment may frequently be needed depending on the person's overall progress and condition, and the intervention adapted based on new assessment/evaluation data.

Activity 10.2 gets you to start thinking about how to evaluate the care and support you provide to others as part of health promotion.

Activity 10.2   Reflection

Reflect on a couple of times when you have been involved in a health promotion intervention with a person. How did you evaluate the intervention? In what way did you measure whether it had been successful or not? How do you think the patient evaluated you and the care and support they received? How do you know this?

Because this is a highly personal activity, there is no outline answer at the end of the chapter. However, you might like to record your answers and reflect on them further while reading the rest of the chapter.

Evaluation of the care and treatment we give is an important aspect of nursing practice. Evaluation is important in healthcare because it supports an evidence-based approach to practice delivery. Consider Activity 10.3.

Activity 10.3   Critical thinking

Patient goals are often, but not always, measured as outcomes (often as SMART goals – specific, measurable, achievable, relevant and timely). Outcome evaluations measure how a person and their circumstances change, as well as whether the treatment experience or intervention has been a factor in causing this change. In other words, outcome evaluations assess treatment effectiveness.

With the permission of your practice supervisor, select several care plans for you to review. Look at how the patient goals are written and then how they are to be evaluated. In pursuing a holistic approach to care, all care plans should include a health promotion activity. It is also worth reflecting on the different approaches used to help the person achieve their goals and the different forms that health promotion takes.

Because the activity is so varied, there is no outline answer at the end of the chapter. However, it could form the basis for an interesting discussion with your supervisor.

When thinking about health promotion, there is a need to recognise that most people have a life beyond and outside of the health service. It is important to remember that patients should be treated as individuals, not as mere objects for processing. Who is the best person to judge whether an intervention has worked or not? The nurse or the person receiving the intervention? A good care plan should be drawn up and actioned in collaboration with the person receiving the intervention and evaluated accordingly.

Conducting a larger-scale evaluation

Is health promotion a good investment? How can the short- and long-term returns of such an investment be assessed? To what degree can social and economic benefits stemming from health promotion initiatives be measured alongside health gains? Answering such questions is not a simple task. Health promotion policies and programmes, if properly planned and implemented, involve complex and sophisticated activities. Often health promotion action requires multiple approaches, relies on interdisciplinary inputs and operates at several levels over long periods of time. How are decisions to be taken and choices made between alternative treatments and interventions, different organisational arrangements and competing strategies? The wide range of evaluative methods that have been developed to date reflect not only the range of questions that need answering, but also the range of activities that require evaluation as part of health promotion. This extends from evaluating a single encounter to that of a complete policy and ways of working. The following section looks at the different types of evaluation, as well as some of the important elements and thinking that need to be addressed when planning a health promotion evaluation. To get you thinking about the complexities involved in planning an evaluation study of a health promotion intervention, consider Activity 10.4.

Activity 10.4   Critical thinking

The Swaffley Foundation School have decided to implement a programme promoting the use of safety helmets while cycling. The scheme has the support of the local council and health service, and the school nurse is actively supporting the programme, highlighting the dangers of having a fall and sustaining a head injury. It is the only secondary school in the town, with only 650 pupils. Below is a brief description of the programme:

Purpose: To increase the use of cycle helmets among 14–18-year-olds in Swaffley and ultimately reduce the number of traumatic head injuries. Helmets were distributed among the pupils and then a campaign created to educate the students on the use and benefits of helmets when riding their bikes – with the school nurse and local police promoting the scheme in class. Pamphlets were also sent home to parents, and a media campaign was launched and promoted through the local newspaper and radio.

Having read the brief description of the programme above, think about the criteria by which you would evaluate whether the scheme had been successful or not.

Compare your answer with the outline answer at the end of the chapter.

Planning

Evaluation requires a great deal of thought and planning if it is to be carried out in the right way for the right reasons. The planning and implementation stages of any health promotion intervention are vital for ensuring successful outcomes. Effective planning and implementation allow staff to look ahead towards the most appropriate evaluation activity (each step informs the other). The planning and implementation phases of a programme of activity, however, are only part of the process, and therefore should always be monitored and followed up by an evaluation phase. Not to do this would in most cases invalidate what had gone previously, as well as providing no real means with which to measure the position, validity, outcomes or success of the programme as it progresses (Lobo et al., 2014).

Most providers do not usually take into account the entire constituent parts of a programme process when planning an activity. It is more likely to be the planning phase that receives the most attention. However, there is a drive to focus on evaluation much earlier in the process in response to the demand to demonstrate the effectiveness of interventions in line with cost (Health Foundation, 2015). Using resources in any activity that produces benefits inevitably involves not using those resources in some other alternative way that would also produce benefits. If we are to compare costs and benefits of different ways of spending scarce healthcare funds, then we need to be able to measure both costs and benefits in such a way that they can be weighted one against the other. This is easier said than done and remains a highly contested area of study.

Concept summary: The principles of health promotion evaluation

In 2001, the WHO European Working Group on Health Promotion met to look at the principles and perspectives of the evaluation of health promotion. The group agreed that health promotion initiatives (programmes, policies and other organised activities) should be:

- empowering (enabling individuals and communities to assume more power over the personal, socioeconomic and environmental factors that affect health);
- participatory (involving all concerned at all stages of the process);
- holistic (fostering physical, mental, social and spiritual health);
- intersectoral (involving the collaboration of agencies from relevant sectors);
- equitable (guided by a concern for equality and social justice);
- sustainable (bringing about changes that individuals and communities can maintain once initial funding has ended);
- multi-strategy (using a variety of approaches – including policy development, organisational change, community development, legislation, advocacy, education and communication – in combination).

(WHO, 2001)

Based on the principles of health promotion, the group concluded that the following are the core features of approaches appropriate for the evaluation of health promotion initiatives.

Participation

At each stage of evaluation, health promotion initiatives should involve, in appropriate ways, those who have a legitimate interest in the initiative. Those with an interest can include policymakers, community members and organisations, health and other professionals and local and national health agencies. It is especially important that members of the community whose health is being addressed be involved in evaluation.

Multiple methods

Evaluations of health promotion initiatives should draw on a variety of disciplines and should consider employing a broad range of information-gathering procedures.

Capacity building

Evaluations of health promotion initiatives should enhance the capacity of individuals, communities, organisations and governments to address important health promotion concerns.

Appropriateness

Evaluations of health promotion initiatives should be designed to accommodate the complex nature of health promotion interventions and their long-term impact.

These guiding principles remain and are reflected in the evaluation of health promotion activities the world over.

There are now a number of **evaluation frameworks** to help the nurse plan and carry out an evaluation. While a degree of variation can be found between these frameworks, they generally contain six broad areas of interest: (1) define your stakeholders; (2) describe the programme or activity to be evaluated; (3) design the evaluation; (4) gather the evidence; (5) draw conclusions based on the evidence generated; and (6) disseminate findings (NWCPHP, 2019). Each of these stages will now be explored. While the process is presented as being linear, it is not unusual to go back and forth between stages as the evaluation progresses.

Step 1: Define your stakeholders

As we have seen from the concept summary above, an essential part of any successful evaluation of a programme or intervention requires engagement with those who have a legitimate interest in the initiative. A stakeholder is anyone who has a stake, or interest, in the evaluation and who may be involved in or affected by it. A stakeholder is either an individual, group or organisation who is said to have a vested interest in what you are doing or proposing. As part of clinical practice, this is likely to be individuals and their families, but could include local community groups and politicians. The level of involvement is often driven by 'how this will impact on me'. Getting stakeholders involved early on will help you get different perspectives on the programme or intervention and establish common expectations. This helps to clarify goals and objectives of the programme or intervention to be evaluated, so everyone understands the need and purpose of the evaluation.

If managed correctly, evaluation has the potential to bring people and groups together and facilitate networking and collaboration. Where practicable, service users and practitioners should be involved throughout the process of evaluation, as it is they who are most likely to be affected by its outcomes. Modern technologies allow involvement over distance, and not all meetings need to be face to face – there should be no excuse for not involving people.

Step 2: Describe the programme or activity to be evaluated

The approach we use to evaluation, the steps you take to evaluate something, will depend on what it is we are being asked to evaluate. This seems self-evident; however, it is not as straightforward as it might seem. Health promotion covers a wide range of activity (see concept summary above), and we need to be able to demonstrate that what we do is having an impact not only on the lives of individuals, but also communities and populations. By definition, health promotion is a process of enabling people to increase control over, and to improve, their health. To be effective, it needs to engage and empower individuals and communities to choose health behaviours and make changes that reduce the risk of developing chronic diseases and other morbidities. These changes usually occur over long periods of time and are often subject to change because of new evidence. This makes outcomes problematic to define, measure and attribute to interventions. Taking the time to articulate what your programme does, as well as what you want to accomplish, is essential to establishing your evaluation plan. The kind of questions that can be answered by evaluation include:

- What is needed? Are we meeting the needs of our users/patients?
- How are people responding to a specific service? Can we improve the programme?
- What happens to our users/patients as a result of following the programme?
- What worked well and what could be done differently next time?
- Are we making the best use of our resources in delivering specific programmes?
- How do costs and benefits compare?
- Are we meeting required standards?

(Marsh and Glendenning, 2005)

Answers to these questions form the basis of evaluation and will assist you in refining your thinking about a programme or intervention, as well as helping you promote the programme or intervention to its beneficiaries. While you might not go on to do an evaluation of a service or intervention on a large scale, the above questions are useful to ask when thinking about the type of care that you are providing.

Step 3: Design the evaluation

An evaluation has to be specifically designed to address the questions being asked and the nature of the intervention being evaluated. Health promotion interventions generally involve a mix of interventions at multiple levels, from the individual through to populations, although single programmes may target only some of these levels. This extends from evaluating a single encounter to that of a complete policy or programme intervention. This means using different methods, working in different settings, with varied populations and data, under specific constraints of time, expertise and resources, both human and financial. The wide range of evaluative techniques available to the clinician reflects not only the range of questions that need answering, but also the range of activities that require evaluation.

There are many types of evaluations to choose from, and it may not always seem clear which one to choose. Evaluation can be broken down into four main categories:

1. formative evaluation;
2. process evaluation;
3. outcome evaluation;
4. impact evaluation.

Concept summary: Types of evaluation

Table 10.2 explores the four main categories of evaluation, along with some more prominent forms of evaluation approaches and the questions they seek to address.

Type	What questions are being asked? The type of question asked will inform the type of evaluation to be undertaken.
Formative assessment	Evaluation processes that are predominantly used to inform programme staff and improve a programme. The goal is to provide feedback on strengths and areas of improvement for the programme, or programme materials, as well as exploring overall applicability and feasibility of the project. Typically takes place prior to programme implementation or early on in the process. Examples: <ul><li>Focus groups with target audience for a programme that is in development at a local community centre.</li><li>A brief 'pen-and-paper' survey of participants in a pilot educational programme on sexual health for teens to understand what programme features they liked and what could be improved.</li><li>One-to-one interviews with current users of a prescription drug to review an informational brochure on medication compliance for content, applicability and ability to produce a call to action.</li></ul>

(Continued)

Table 10.2 (Continued)

Process evaluation	How is the policy implemented? Do we observe expected behaviours? Why or why not? Process evaluations look at how the programme has been delivered and the processes by which it was implemented. A process evaluation may be conducted periodically throughout the life of the programme or to look back over the programme. It may help to explain why a programme did or did not meet its main objectives. The goal is to examine how the programme was implemented. Examples: • Assess what percentage of parents in an online course about talking to your teen about drugs fully completed the online education module. • Interview programme co-ordinators about internal procedures for training healthcare providers on new guidelines for a hospital-based screening programme targeted at identifying the early warning signs of psychosis in their patient population.
Outcome/ impact evaluation	Did the programme produce the intended effects compared to what would have happened anyway? It can help understand 'what works' and can then be useful to understand whether this will work for different groups in different settings. Outcome evaluation data are often used to determine if the programme should be adopted, expanded or continued. Was the programme effective? Did it meet the objective(s)? The goal is to determine whether outcomes observed are due to the programme. Examples: • *Randomised control trial example.* For a new peer mentor programme at a local health centre to increase percentage of TB patients who are compliant with their medication regimens, randomly half were selected to receive a new programme with one-to-one peer mentoring, while the other half received the standard discussion with their provider and an informational brochure. • *Quasi-experimental example.* A time series design to explore the impact of a new sexual education course within a school district on teen pregnancy. Data on teen pregnancy rates were collected for five years prior and five years after programme implementation to see if rates changed post-programme initiation.

Cost-benefit analysis	Are the policy benefits worth the costs? Cost-benefit analysis looks to understand all the results from the data that have been gathered. It makes estimations about the strengths and weaknesses of an approach and monetises this to see whether the costs are worth paying for the benefits received.
Monitoring	Is the implementation progressing as planned?
Performance management	Performance management is a more formalised process of monitoring to ensure that objectives and milestones are being reached in an efficient and effective way.

Table 10.2   The four main categories of evaluation

In addition to being focused on formative, process or outcome, evaluations can be:

- *prospective*: designed before the programme has been implemented;
- *retrospective*: designed and conducted after a programme has been implemented.

(CDC, 2011)

As you begin formulating your evaluation, think about the specific purpose of the evaluation. What questions are you trying to answer? How will the information be used? What information-gathering methods are best suited for collecting what your organisation needs to know?

Step 4: Gather the evidence

Conceptually, evaluation research promotes the value of utilising knowledge from different sources to form a cohesive whole and will depend on the type of evaluation being undertaken. The most commonly used methods of data collection in evaluation include document analysis, surveys, interviews, observations, focus groups and case studies. These can be qualitative, quantitative or both. Qualitative data offer descriptive information that may capture experience, behaviour, opinion, value, feeling, knowledge, sensory response or observable phenomena and seek to understand the 'lived experience' of those involved in the intervention or programme. Three commonly used methods used for gathering qualitative evaluation data are key informant interviews, focus groups and participant observation. Quantitative methods refer to information that may be measured by numbers or tallies. Methods for collecting quantitative data include counting systems (e.g. counting how many times a person completes a certain activity), surveys and questionnaires.

Step 5: Draw conclusions based on the evidence generated

For any evaluation, drawing conclusions based on the evidence is the most important part of the process. Your conclusions should be based solely on what you found. Data analysis involves identifying and summarising the key findings, themes and information contained in data generated by the evaluation (Linsley et al., 2019). You can compare evaluation data with targets set for the programme against standards established by your stakeholders or funders, or make comparisons with other programmes.

Step 6: Disseminate findings

It is important that all the work you put into programme evaluation gets used for quality improvement and moving practice forward. The dissemination of health promotion evaluation findings is crucial in establishing a strong evidence base for health promotion. You need to document not only what worked, but what did not, as well as possible reasons for success and failure (Round et al., 2005). When you present your findings and recommendations, it is important to know the values, beliefs and perceptions of your group, to build on the group's background and common ground and to state the underlying purpose for your recommendations before you get to the details. A mix of dissemination strategies can be used, including:

- feeding into the training of staff;
- communication through print, including summary reports for different audiences and peer-reviewed journal articles (where possible, publication of the results in a peer-reviewed journal is encouraged and supported by the department to contribute to the health promotion evidence base);
- communication through ICTs, platforms and social media;
- personal face-to-face contacts, including briefings and presentations, journal clubs and clinical handovers;
- policies, administrative arrangements and funding incentives.

Above all, it is important to celebrate successes, something that we do not do enough.

Evaluation, monitoring and clinical audit

Evaluation is sometimes confused between monitoring, clinical audit and evaluation. While there is some overlap between these activities, they are in fact different. Monitoring is a process of observing and checking in to see if things are going to plan. This may involve collecting, analysing and using information to track progress. Once the value of an activity has been demonstrated and generally accepted as worthwhile, you only need to evaluate periodically. There is, however, a need for continuous monitoring to assess first whether or not the activity is being implemented, and second, even if it is, that it is achieving the results expected from the initial evaluation. Furthermore, establishing the value of some aspect of healthcare does not guarantee that either an individual or society at large will benefit from its use. Take two examples:

1. Antibiotics have been shown to be effective in a carefully designed study, but in general use they might be prescribed too frequently or not frequently enough.

2. A particular diet might have evaluated well, but this does not guarantee it will be widely adopted, owing to it being costly.

In this sense, evaluation is not enough. It is also necessary to monitor services and activity to see whether or not we are providing the best possible services and care within resources to the benefit of those that use the service, the patient and the general public. For instance, when assessing the impact of a policy, it may be necessary to both evaluate and monitor it while it is being implemented. Clinical audit would be an example of this. Clinical audit involves assessment of practice against criteria derived from evidence and standards based on published performance, previous achievement or consensus, with the aim of implementing change to bring about improvement. Audit requires the measurement of care (how we are doing) against established criteria and standards (what we should be doing) against which performance can be measured. The audit cycle requires change to be implemented for improvements (how we can improve on what we are doing) in performance to occur (how the changes we have made have led to improvement). It is usually specific to the site and time at which it was carried out, although larger regional, national or multinational audits are limited in what they measure (e.g. response times from referral to seeing a patient) (Harding and Jarvis, 2019). There are many websites and resources to support you when thinking of undertaking an evaluation. The following activity takes you to one such highly creditable site.

Activity 10.5   Critical thinking

Visit the Evaluation Works website, which is supported by the National Institute for Health Research: **www.nhsevaluationtoolkit.net/resources/case-studies/**

The site contains a number of case studies that have been developed to illustrate how evaluation can be used to inform decision making. Take time to explore the site, clicking on each of the headers, which contain an abundance of information. Take time to look at each case study and how the different parties went about conducting their evaluation. Make notes as you go as to the key elements that stand out for you, as well as what you might like to explore in greater depth going forward in your studies.

As this activity focuses on you, there is no outline answer at the end of the chapter.

Chapter summary

In its broadest sense, evaluation is a systematic process to understand what a programme or activity does and how well it does it. The first step in undertaking an evaluation, as with any research study, whether of your care or practice, service or policy, is to clarify the purpose of evaluation. It is important that you understand what the need for the evaluation is and what is driving it. There is a need to determine whether services and health promotion interventions are of the highest quality (i.e. safe, effective, efficient) and geared to enhancing the patient experience by being timely, accessible and patient centred. An evaluation project can support any of the following three aims:

1. support the development of your activity (formative evaluation);
2. ensure you manage it better next time (evaluation of your processes);
3. assess the final impact of your activity (summative evaluation).

When conducted properly, evaluation aspires to be systematic and rigorous, just as research and audit, and it may use similar methods of quantitative or qualitative data collection and analysis. Above all, health promotion interventions are complex; their evaluation requires a lot of planning and co-ordination, time and effort. Having done all this and completed the evaluation, it is important that you disseminate the findings and celebrate its successes.

Activities: Brief outline answers

Activity 10.1   Critical thinking (page 156)

You may carry out an evaluation of the care that you give for personal reasons, such as continuing professional development, **revalidation** or simply out of individual interest and for individual growth borne out of curiosity. You may have been asked to evaluate a service or health promotion activity to demonstrate its usefulness, for marketing to service users or for commissioners, deciding whether to continue with the current approaches, or when considering whether to design or purchase new models of provision.

Activity 10.4   Critical thinking (page 159)

There is a number of ways in which you could judge the merits of the scheme and whether the scheme had been successful or not. For example, what percentage of students, having received in-class instruction on helmet use, then started wearing a helmet when riding their bike? Did the incident of brain injury from cycle accidents among 14–18-year-olds following the distribution of helmets go down? (Swaffley is only a small rural town of 7,500 people, with no reported head injuries from a cycling accident in the last five years, and only one in the last ten years.) What percentage of parents read the pamphlets sent home with their child and then took steps to ensure that their child always wore a helmet when out riding their bike? A measure of success could be that 90 per cent of students were still wearing helmets six months after the scheme finished, two years after the scheme finished, or 20 years after the scheme finished.

Often when we start to look at evaluation in terms of success, it throws up more questions than it answers. Using our example, the wearing of helmets is not as straightforward as it seems. Helmets have been proven to be effective in reducing injuries; however, the effectiveness of the helmet is dependent on the type of collision in which the cyclist is involved, the injury tolerance of the rider and the surface with which the helmet makes contact (e.g. kerb, car bonnet) (Forbes et al., 2017). Interestingly, the Royal Society for the Prevention of Accidents does not support calls for compulsory cycle helmet laws because it is not clear whether such a law would discourage some people from cycling, which, if it did, would mean losing the health and environmental benefits from cycling (ROSPA, 2018).

Further reading

WHO (2001) *Evaluation in Health Promotion: Principles and Perspectives.* WHO Regional Publication Series, No. 92.

Despite being published in 2001, this WHO publication remains a key text for those interested in the evaluation of health promotion.

Useful websites

www.betterevaluation.org/en

An international collaboration to improve evaluation practice and theory by sharing and generating information about evaluation methods, processes and approaches.

www.cdc.gov/eval/steps/index.htm

This provides a framework for programme evaluation based on six steps. Especially helpful are activities and checklists that you can download as PDFs for use in practice.

www.gov.uk/guidance/evaluation-in-health-and-wellbeing-introduction

This Government UK website provides an introduction to evaluation in health and well-being and provides further links to related content. Well worth exploring.

Chapter 11 Promoting one's own health

Chapter aims

After reading this chapter, you will be able to:

- understand how what you eat, how active you are and how decisions you make about your behaviour and relationships affect your physical and mental well-being;
- participate in a range of activities that promote a healthy lifestyle;
- reflect on your strengths and skills to help make informed choices when thinking about your own health and well-being.

Introduction

Being a nurse brings its own demands and challenges. Workplace conditions, as well as the stress of dealing with vulnerable people on a daily basis, can take a toll on your physical health and emotional well-being. This situation has been made worse by the COVID-19 pandemic and the tremendous demand and strain this has put on staff and students. As we transition to living and working alongside COVID-19 and start to tackle the backlog of work, it's more important than ever to look after ourselves and manage our demands accordingly. Consider the following quote from Dr Anna Baverstock of Somerset NHS Foundation Trust:

> *In order to provide compassionate, safe and high-quality care, staff well-being is paramount. We cannot expect to look after others if we don't look after ourselves and our teams …. Using the analogy of a phone battery that drains and needs recharging is how I like to think about each aspect of well-being. We often are aware when our phone is on red and needs to be plugged in but how often do we do a battery check for our own personal reveres?*

(HEE, 2019b, page 51)

The message is a simple one: you need to look after your own health in order to look after the health of others. It is important to 'keep charging the battery' and to make sure that 'you don't run flat'.

The following chapter is designed to help you think about your own health and well-being. It starts by looking at ways to maintain good health and well-being when going about your duties as a nurse. The chapter then looks at the signs and symptoms of caregivers' stress and burnout, as well as how students might go about building resilience to these. The chapter ends with a summary of the key points and provides links to self-care resources.

Getting started

Shift work, stress, heavy workloads and the emotional labour of nursing can make it particularly difficult for nurses to make healthy lifestyle choices. Nurses will often put the needs of their patients before their own. The COVID-19 crisis has undoubtedly had an impact on the mental health and well-being of nurses due to the increase of occupational psychosocial risks, such as emotional exhaustion and work-related stress levels. During the height of COVID-19 we saw nurses and other healthcare professionals having to choose between the health of their patients and that of their own and family's health. Many nurses did not go home between shifts fearing the spread of infection but instead chose to isolate in quickly repurposed staff accommodation.

As a nurse, it is important that you take the time to consider factors that impact upon your own health and well-being, as well as those that you care for and look after. We need to become self-caring. Self-care relates to any action that improves, develops, protects or maintains your overall health and well-being, and it starts with the individual responsibility people take in making daily choices about their lifestyle, such as brushing their teeth, eating healthily or choosing to walk or bike to work. Make no mistake, nursing is an incredibly rewarding and worthwhile career; however, it is not without its challenges and demands. With a busy workload, it can often feel impossible to delegate 'me time'; however, you would be surprised how much even the smallest of lifestyle changes can contribute towards improving your overall wellness. Complete Activities 11.1 and 11.2 before going on and reading the rest of the chapter.

Activity 11.1   Reflection

How many of these have you experienced in clinical practice?

- Missing your break or taking your break late because you are focused on making sure your patient is safe and comfortable.
- Walking around with a full bladder because you were too busy to go to the toilet.
- Staying late after a shift to fill out paperwork you did not have time to do during the day.
- Not getting a good night's sleep between a late and early shift.
- Eating unhealthy food because you are too tired after a shift to prepare a healthy meal.
- Doing extra shifts on the bank and not being able to spend time with your loved ones.
- Not having enough time to process things seen on shift.
- Not having the energy or the time to participate in regular exercise.

The chances are that you will relate to some, if not all, of the above. All are indicators that you are putting your health and well-being at risk. Now reflect on some of the ways you might go about addressing the issues highlighted.

An outline answer with a few suggestions on how you might go about tackling some of these issues raised in the activity is provided at the end of the chapter.

Activity 11.2   Reflection

To begin to improve your physical and mental well-being, it is important to spend time carrying out a self-care assessment. Trying to force self-care into your lifestyle without a goal or an objective becomes a limiting exercise. Start by asking yourself the following questions:

- How much downtime do you have a week?
- Do you eat a balanced diet?
- Do you get enough sleep?

- What activities do you participate in outside of work?
- How often do you socialise with friends and family?
- Are you able to pursue a hobby?
- When did you last do something for yourself?

Because this is a personal reflective exercise, there is no outline answer at the end of the chapter.

Looking after our own health and well-being

'Taking care of your basic needs' means making sure you look after yourself and your health, as well as eating and sleeping well. This means knowing what your body needs and what will keep you rested, well and strong. Four main factors emerge from the literature when thinking about looking after yourself: eating well and taking on plenty of fluids, taking part in some form of physical activity, spending quality time with family and friends, and resting and sleeping well (RCN, 2019). These four factors will now be explored in greater depth.

Eating well

One of the 'hazards' of working in a healthcare team is that meal breaks can take place at unusual and unpredictable times. Some nurses will work through their breaks because they do not feel that they can leave the clinical area; others will simply forget that they have not had a break because they are so caught up in their work. How many times have you heard a nurse say, 'Where's the time gone?'

Always ensure that, even on the busiest of days, you always take your break and never opt for skipping meals. Skipping meals forces your body into 'fasting mode', meaning that your blood glucose levels will begin to drop. Your blood glucose levels are your brain's main source of fuel; a lack of glucose will immediately start to impact on your concentration levels and motivation, as well as increasing fatigue. Food is fuel, and you need to make sure that you get the right amount, at the right time, of the right sort.

Aim to have a balanced diet. A balanced diet is one consisting of a variety of different types of food and providing adequate amounts of the nutrients necessary for good health (NHS, 2019e). A problem with nurses and a number of people in general is that they will snack and eat junk food rather than prepare a proper meal. Try to have fewer foods and drinks that are high in fat, salt and sugars. Instead, try to choose a variety of foods high in fibre, vitamins and minerals, such as fruit, vegetables and wholegrains. Consider snacking on carrot strips, fruit bars or indeed a piece of fruit. Not only is this good for weight control; it is also good for your heart (Heart Foundation, 2019).

Meal breaks are not just about eating your food but taking time away from the stresses and strains of work. One of the most effective ways to ensure that you are never forced to skip meals is to prep your lunch break snack in advance. Spend time the evening before your shift putting together a tasty, nutritious meal that you can grab from the fridge on your way out the door. Try to enjoy your food and take time to eat it properly. Eating your meals quickly can lead to indigestion but can also add to the feeling of being under pressure. Take your time eating; those five minutes relaxing chewing your food could be the energy boost that you need.

Last but not least, do not forget to treat yourself to food that makes you feel good. While, of course, it is important to stay healthy, you also need to be realistic. If that delicious piece of lemon cheesecake in the staff canteen is staring you in the eye, go for it! Looking after yourself is also about looking after your mental health. A little bit of what you fancy does you good every now and then.

Take on plenty of fluids – stay hydrated

Although we are all more than aware of the importance of drinking water, we have all at times likely fallen guilty of going hours on end without any form of hydration. It is important to keep hydrated or our health can suffer. Nearly two-thirds of your body is water, which means that it is a vital source of energy to survive. Water helps you digest your food, absorb nutrients from food and then get rid of the unused waste through urination, perspiration and bowel movements. In the UK, the NHS recommends consuming six to eight glasses a day, or 1.9 litres (almost 34 fl oz), including water that is in food. However, the amount of water we need depends on individual needs and circumstances, including activity and climate, and such measures should serve as a guide rather than an absolute.

There are many different ways in which you can encourage yourself to drink more water each day, including using a marked water bottle. You can now get bottles printed with each hour of the day to mark your progress. A marked water bottle is ideal for visually keeping track of how much water you have drunk throughout the day, as well as serving as a visual reminder to drink more.

There are now many different free apps that send notifications to your mobile to remind you to drink water (e.g. Daily Water Tracker Reminder for iPhone, Hydro Coach for Android). These allow you to log how many glasses of water you drink each time to ensure that you reach your daily target. Reflect on Activity 11.3.

Activity 11.3   Reflection

The Quench has a guide to the ten best apps available to monitor your daily water intake, a number of which are free: **www.thequench.com/water/8-of-the-best-water-apps-to-use-for-free/**

Take the time to visit the site, and if keeping hydrated is a problem, then consider downloading an app.

Because this is a matter for you to decide on, there is no outline answer at the end of the chapter.

If you are less keen on the thought of drinking fresh water, there is no harm in adding a fruity twist. Lemon, berries and grapefruit are all ideal for adding flavour to your water. You could even consider purchasing a fruit infuser water bottle. If you prefer hot drinks, try experimenting with swapping your mid-morning coffee for a fruity or peppermint tea.

Case study: Taking on fluids

Student nurse Hayley Miles has decided that she needs to take on more fluids during the course of her working day. As well as getting a water tracker, Hayley and her friend, student nurse Jane Day, who is on the same placement as Hayley, will remind each other to take on fluids as they pass in the corridor. This has acted as a real motivator for Hayley, and she finds that she is drinking more.

Physical activity

People are less active nowadays, partly because technology has made our lives easier. We drive cars or take public transport. Work, household chores, shopping and other necessary activities are far less demanding than for previous generations. However, it is never too late to get active. Any physical activity for ten or more minutes that is of at least moderate intensity (i.e. raises your breathing rate) is beneficial to health (DHSC, 2019). To stay healthy, adults should try to be active every day and aim to achieve at least 150 minutes of physical activity over a week through a variety of activities. For most people, the easiest way to get moving is to make activity part of everyday life, such as walking or cycling instead of using the car to get around. The more exercise you do, the better, and taking part in activities such as sports will make you even healthier. However, you need to strike a balance, and not overdo it and cause yourself an injury. As with all things, everything in moderation.

For any type of activity to benefit your health, you need to be moving quick enough to raise your heart rate, breathe faster and feel warmer. This is called moderate activity. An activity where you have to work even harder is called vigorous-intensity activity. There is substantial evidence that vigorous-intensity activity can bring health benefits over and above that of moderate activity. You can tell when it is vigorous activity because you are breathing hard and fast and your heart rate has gone up quite a bit. If you are working at this level, you would not be able to say more than a few words without pausing for a breath (NHS, 2019a). Choose exercise activities you enjoy. Not only are you more likely to stick with them, but you also avoid the negative effects of forcing yourself to do something you dislike. There are many available options, such as walking, running, swimming and cycling, which are relatively inexpensive.

Finally, think about activities you could co-ordinate with your caring role, or do with the person you care for to help keep you both active. For example, within mental health, would it not be good to get people off the ward and to go for a walk? As a clinician, Paul, one of the authors, used to run a gardening club, and the mental health trust provided a small garden that he and service users would tend. As well as gaining exercise by digging the plot, it proved to be a good way to promote socialisation and communication.

Case study: Increasing physical activity

As part of her 'fitness drive', student nurse Hayley Miles has decided to take on more physical exercise. As part of this, Hayley no longer takes the lift at work, but instead uses the stairs. This small measure has had real benefits. Hayley has found that it has built up her aerobic capacity and muscle strength. She has also noticed that there is a minimal time difference between using the lift and the stairs. It is also another way that Hayley gets her steps in for the day.

Spending quality time with family and friends

It is important that you try to keep up your social connections as these are good for maintaining your own well-being (NHS Inform, 2019), particularly those with family and friends – even if it is just a quick phone call or Skype. The health benefits of spending time with friends and family can extend to every part of a person's life. Loved ones can encourage positive behaviours, such as taking more exercise, eating healthily or cutting down on your alcohol intake, as well as discouraging negative behaviours such as smoking.

Another one of the health benefits of spending time with friends and family is improved mental health. Social interaction and mental health have long been linked together for having a cause-and-effect relationship. Face-to-face contact can reduce the risk of mental illness, such as depression and anxiety. It is no secret that confiding in your friends and family is a healthy way to relieve stress. Texting and social media are no substitution for spending time with friends and family. Being surrounded by a supportive network of people can help you to build confidence and maintain healthy self-esteem.

Concept summary: Social contact

Five things you can do:

1. *Give time.* Put more time aside to connect with friends and family.
2. *Be present.* It can be tempting to check your phone, Facebook messages or even work e-mails when with family and friends. Try to be present in the moment and be there for your loved ones and switch to out-of-work mode whenever possible.

---

3. *Listen*: Actively listen to what others are saying in a non-judgemental way and concentrate on their needs in that moment.
4. *Be listened to*: Share how you are feeling, honestly, and allow yourself to be listened to and supported.
5. *Recognise unhealthy relationships*: Being around positive people can make us happier; however, our well-being can be negatively affected by harmful relationships, leaving us unhappy. Recognising this can help us move forward and find solutions to issues.

(Mental Health Foundation, 2019)

It is also important to note that family and friend groups can also encourage continued unhealthy behaviours, and individuals may need to seek support from elsewhere to break old habits. Instead, find someone who will be a positive influence, whether they are someone you know personally or a positive role model in the public eye. Help to change your mindset by using positive words in your day-to-day conversations.

Resting well – getting enough sleep

Get the rest you need. This is not always easy, but stress can get worse when sleep deprivation takes hold, and your motivation will decrease if you feel tired and drained. Sleep and health are strongly related – poor sleep can increase the risk of having poor health, and poor health can make it harder to sleep. Sleep disturbances can be one of the first signs of distress. Common mental health problems such as anxiety and depression can often underpin sleep problems. Sleep is especially challenging in shift-based work and safety-critical industries such as health, so it is even more important to make sure we get the right amount of good-quality sleep if we are to safeguard our practice.

It is easy to think about sleep as a time when your body and brain temporarily shut off. The truth, however, is that during rest, your brain is hard at work overseeing a wide variety of biological upkeep and preparing for the next day. It is important that you get a good night's sleep. Good sleep allows you to prepare for the next day by helping your mind to regain focus and ready itself to tackle those tricky mental challenges. It is no surprise that we are unable to concentrate and apply ourselves to tasks when we are feeling tired and run-down. It can also stimulate creativity and boost memory. Sleeping is the most important time to shape memories and make the connections between events, feelings and experiences. In fact, sleep is a requirement to form new learning and memory pathways in the brain.

Sleep also allows the body to repair itself and fight off infection. When you do not get enough, your immune system is weaker, making you more susceptible to illness. During sleep, your body repairs the damage caused by stress, ultraviolet rays and other harmful exposure, as well as muscle injuries and other traumas, including mental trauma. Furthermore, energy levels after healthy sleep are higher and your mental awareness is more acute (RSPH, 2019).

We can all benefit from improving the quality of our sleep. For many of us, it may simply be a case of making small lifestyle or attitude adjustments in order to help us sleep better. Preparing for sleep, or sleep hygiene, should be an important part of your daily routine. Winding down is a critical stage in preparing for bed. There are lots of ways to relax and promote sleep following a long shift. A warm bath (not hot) can help your body to reach a temperature that is ideal for rest and relaxation. Reflecting on the day and writing 'to-do' lists for the next day can help to organise your thoughts and clear your mind of distractions. It also helps to foster a feeling of being in control, something that is important for good mental health.

Take time to relax before going to sleep and perhaps enjoy a relaxing hot drink. Try listening to soft music and/or reading a bedtime story, although not from an e-reader, which can heighten brain activity. Likewise, avoid using smartphones, tablets or other electronic devices for an hour or so before you go to bed, as the light from the screen on these devices may have a negative effect on sleep (NHS, 2019b).

Make your bedroom sleep friendly. Your bedroom should be a relaxing environment. Experts claim that there is a strong association in people's minds between sleep and the bedroom (NHS, 2019b). However, certain things weaken that association, such as TVs and other electronic gadgets, light, noise and a bad mattress or bed. Your bedroom ideally needs to be dark, quiet, tidy and be kept at a temperature of between 18°C and 24°C. Fit some thick curtains if you do not have any. If you are disturbed by noise, consider using earplugs.

Most adults need between six and nine hours of sleep every night. By working out what time you need to wake up, you can set a regular bedtime schedule. It is also important to try to wake up at the same time every day if you can. While it may seem like a good idea to try to 'catch up' on sleep after a bad night, doing so on a regular basis can also disrupt your sleep routine. There are a number of apps designed to help with sleep (see the NHS Apps Library in the useful websites section at the end of the chapter).

Case study: Getting to sleep

Student nurse Hayley Miles has had trouble switching off and getting to sleep between a late and an early shift. She lives in shared accommodation near to a main road, which can be noisy at times. Hayley tried wearing earplugs but did not get on with these. What she did instead was create a calming playlist of music on her mobile phone, and she plays this at low volume when she goes to bed. The music helps her to relax and blocks out a lot of the background noise that used to distract her. It has now become part of her sleep routine. Hayley seldom finds that she gets past the fifth song before she has fallen asleep.

Stress and building resilience for health and well-being

Stress can affect anyone, but the pressure and expectations of caring can make nurses particularly vulnerable. Under normal circumstances people's reactions to stress should enable them to find new balances and responses to new situations. Stress is therefore not necessarily a negative phenomenon but can act to motivate a person to try out new ideas and ways of working, as well as to move practice forward. Some stress, therefore, is normal and necessary. However, if stress is intense, continuous or repeated, if the person is unable to cope or if support is lacking, as we saw during COVID-19, then stress can become a negative phenomenon leading to physical illness and psychological disorders. A very common issue that you may have heard about is burnout (see Table 11.1). This occurs when immense pressure is put on to a person, culminating in 'chronic stress'. That stress could be caused by a variety of things, from outrageous workloads (and no work–life balance) to simply not feeling valued for the hard work you do.

Concept summary: Burnout

Common signs and symptoms of stress among caregivers	Common signs and symptoms of caregiver burnout
• Anxiety, depression, irritability	• You have much less energy than you once had
• Feeling tired and run down	• It seems like you catch every cold or bout of flu that is going around
• Difficulty sleeping	• You are constantly exhausted, even after sleeping or taking a break
• Overreacting to minor nuisances	• You neglect your own needs, either because you are too busy, or you do not care any more
• New or worsening health problems	• Your life revolves around caregiving, but it gives you little satisfaction
• Trouble concentrating	• You have trouble relaxing, even when help is available
• Feeling increasingly resentful	• You are increasingly impatient and irritable with the person that you are caring for
• Drinking, smoking or eating more	• You feel helpless and hopeless
• Neglecting responsibilities	• Not meeting expectations
• Cutting back on leisure activities	• Isolating oneself

Table 11.1   Common signs and symptoms of stress and caregiver burnout

If you do notice that you have been acting out of character lately, then it may be time to start assessing your work–life balance. For many people, achieving a good quality of life is dependent on striking a balance between the demands of employment and their responsibilities outside work. Work–life balance can be defined as having sufficient control and autonomy over where, when and how you work to fulfil your responsibilities within and outside paid work (RCN, 2017). Some argue for the phrase 'life–work' balance to be used instead as it seeks to address the imbalance between work and home demands.

Having the time to devote to your life outside of work means you are better able to cope with pressures in the workplace. One of the first steps in dealing with stress is to acknowledge that it is happening and to think about the reasons. Starting to deal with the causes, even by taking very small steps, helps you feel more in control. The earlier you do this, the better. Just talking about how you feel with someone can help you find a way to deal with it. Another way of dealing with the stresses and strains of life is building resilience to them.

Social media and stress

Social media have many benefits, but unfortunately everything in this world has its negative sides. Despite the many advantages associated with social media, there are a number of negative effects caused by their usage. Among the common negative effects of social media use are stress, anxiety, depression and addiction. Social media are great for keeping up to date with things and staying in touch with family and friends, but they can become all-consuming and take over people's lives. Despite all the mentioned effects of social media, we can cope without them. All we need is to know how to use them in a healthy way. One of the ways to reduce stress induced by social media is reducing the time we spend on them. Use social media with an intention other than having to pass time.

Concept summary: The end of the 'mindless scroll'

Cal Newport (2019), an associate professor of computer science at Georgetown University, has developed a practical guide to help us use our devices with intention and end the 'mindless scroll'. He suggests the following five ways to digital detox, training yourself to pick up your device when you need it, the 'meaningful scroll':

1. *Cold turkey*: Give up all personal social media accounts for 30 days.
2. *Night owl*: Take a break from the internet every evening after 6 p.m.
3. *Social butterfly*: Switch off your phone and tablet at all social events.
4. *Busy bee*: Take a break from personal social media accounts when you are at work.
5. *Sleeping dog*: Keep any screens out of your bedroom to improve sleep.

Building resilience

Resilience is the ability to cope under pressure and recover from difficulties. A person who has good resilience copes well under pressure and can bounce back more quickly than someone whose resilience is less developed. Being resilient will help you to manage stressful situations, protect you from mental ill health and improve your health and well-being. At work, this ensures that you can continue to do your job well, as well as delivering high-quality care and support. It can also support you in your personal life. Resilient people benefit from better job satisfaction as they are more able to cope with the stress and demands of work, which in turn can lead to better personal and professional working relationships (Skills for Care, 2019).

When we are resilient, we not only adapt ourselves to stress and disappointments; we also grow the insight to avoid actions that might lead us to face such situations. Being resilient is about being able to withstand setbacks, frustrations and personal tragedies. During a crisis, the resilient person will do their best to cope with events calmly, with grace, patience, acceptance and hope. The less resilient person might respond with anger, fear, frustration and impatience, as well as seeing themselves as the victim.

Activity 11.4   Reflection

The following are behaviours associated with resilience. How many of the behaviours would you say relate to you?

- Understanding and valuing the meaning of what you do. Build self-esteem by reminding yourself of your strengths and qualities. Try to replace negative thoughts about a problem with positive ones.
- Greeting new situations, people and demands with a positive attitude. Try to be as flexible as possible in the face of change. Sudden changes, in particular, can seem very disruptive. Try, wherever possible, to see positives in the change.
- Doing what you can to get on with other people.
- Taking a problem-solving approach to difficulty. Experiment with and use a range of problem-solving strategies. Set reasonable goals to deal with problems. Break problem solving down into small manageable steps.
- Keeping a sense of perspective (and humour) when things go wrong.
- Being flexible and willing to adapt to change.
- Drawing on a range of strategies to cope with pressure. A resilient person can recognise when pressure is causing them a problem. Healthcare is a stressful environment in which to work. Having mechanisms in place to cope will help you develop resilience and protect your own mental health.
- Taking action to solve problems as soon as they are encountered. The problem is probably not going to go away, and the longer you leave it, the more stressed you will feel.

(Continued)

(Continued)

- Recognising your thoughts and emotions and managing them.
- Asking for help when you need it. Maintain a supportive social network of nursing colleagues. Talk to them about problems and make use of your combined experiences.
- Being willing to persevere when the going gets tough.
- Recognising and respecting your own limits, including what you can control and what you cannot.

(Skills for Care, 2019)

Given the personal nature of this activity, there is no outline answer at the end of the chapter. However, you might like to look at the list and see what behaviours you could adopt going forward as part of your work and everyday life. Any change can only be for the positive.

A resilient person has a sense of purpose and direction to their life. They are self-aware and have insight into the way they think and behave. Through self-awareness, we gain a deeper understanding of how feelings contribute to our actions. Rather than looking for help outside or blaming the world for our unhappiness, self-awareness gives us the courage to look for answers within ourselves. By making us more attuned to our inner world, building self-awareness helps us to become more capable and cognisant.

When faced with a challenging situation, being aware of what has led to it can help you change your behaviour to take a different path next time. You may feel you did not handle a certain situation well, or perhaps a patient or their family member became angry for some reason. There are many different sides and perspectives to a situation, and all sides and experiences can be valid. A resilient person has strategies to cope with both in-the-moment and long-term pressure.

People with higher levels of emotional and self-control can redirect themselves and manipulate their feelings. They are less likely to be overwhelmed by stress or let it affect their lives. They think before taking the leap and will not surge fast into drawing conclusions. Above all, remember that many problems nurses face in their daily work are the result of organisational weaknesses or failures. Try not to feel responsible for situations that are beyond your control. Having good personal relationships is both a by-product and a requisite for resilience. Ultimately, for nurses, building resilience is a form of self-care that will benefit both yourself and your patients.

Concept summary: Realistic optimism

Developing positive thinking and realistic optimism are important components to resilience. Realistic optimism means seeing things as they are accurately, then making the best of them to maintain a positive outlook while being aware of the difficulties that exist.

People who are optimistic tend to be happier and more able to cope when times get tough. However, it is also possible to be unrealistically positive if you pretend things are fine when they are not.

Consider this idea: The things we can change, we should. The things we cannot change, we must accept.

Realistic optimism is not about unrealistic wishful thinking, and it is certainly not about ignoring problems. Realistic optimism is about engaging with life positively and constructively, taking personal responsibility for your choices, taking a problem-solving approach to difficulty and looking for positive solutions (Skills for Care, 2019).

Mindfulness

Mindfulness has been promoted as another component of resilience. The essence of mindfulness can be summed up in three words: 'be here now'. Paying more attention to the present moment – to your own thoughts and feelings, and to the world around you – can improve your mental well-being. Mindfulness involves paying full attention to your feelings, thoughts and bodily sensations in the present moment. This means standing aside from any other thoughts, worries, upsets and plans that normally absorb and preoccupy your mind. It is easy to stop noticing the world around us and lose touch with what our body is telling us. Being mindful enables you to disengage from your worries and upsets, give yourself some distance from everyday stress and regain perspective and a deeper sense of self. The key to mindfulness is learning how to pay attention.

Mindfulness can take place through meditation sessions or smaller moments throughout the day. To cultivate a state of mindfulness, you can begin by sitting down and taking deep breaths. Focus on each breath and the sensations of the moment, such as sounds, scents, the temperature and the feeling of air passing in and out of the body.

Then shift your attention to the thoughts and emotions that you are experiencing. Allow each thought to exist without judging it or ascribing negativity to it. Sit with those thoughts. The experience may evoke a strong emotional reaction. Exploring that response can be an opportunity to address or resolve underlying challenges.

Who to go to for help?

Seeking help and support is a sign of strength, not a weakness. Never feel as if you are going it alone. If tasks are beginning to build up, stress levels are rising and you are starting to feel the strain, do not keep it to yourself. Talking with others is one of the best forms of self-care.

If you are feeling overwhelmed, stressed or troubled by something in clinical practice, then you can always talk to your supervisor or the nurse in charge. Your supervisor is the person who most understands your training and the demands of your practice environment. Likewise, your university will offer a range of pastoral and academic support, and it is important to access this earlier rather than later, not letting things bubble away, but seeking help when it is required.

As a student, it is also important to remember that you have access to student support services. Student support services offer a range of professional, proactive and approachable services for students dependent on individual need. This includes such things as support with finances, life advice and counselling, occupational health services and study support.

Activity 11.5   Talking about your own and others' mental health: Positive action

We don't do enough talking about our mental health. The LetsShare Campaign was a campaign run by Cardiff University and was developed in collaboration with the Time to Change (2018) movement. The campaign helped students and staff to talk safely about their mental health and well-being without fear of stigmatisation and repercussion and contained five key messages. These were:

1. Speak about your mental health
2. Help others to talk about their mental health
3. Access support for mental health
4. Recognise that the language we use to talk about mental health is important
5. Expect small things to make a big difference.

Explore the campaign further by visiting the campaign website using the following link: https://blogs.cardiff.ac.uk/mental-health/letsshare/

Also visit the Time to Change website: https://www.time-to-change.org.uk/about-us/ Time to Change was a social movement to change the way people think and act when it comes to mental health problems. The campaign started in 2007 and closed at the end of March 2021. It was the largest such campaign run in the UK and it's interesting to read what they did and what they achieved through their work.

You may also want to visit the Act Belong Commit Campaign in Western Australia, which is aimed at getting people to talk about their mental health:

https://www.actbelongcommit.org.au/

Chapter summary

Although nurses are trained caregivers, they sometimes forget the importance of self-care. This can lead to errors on the job, fatigue, burnout and poor physical and mental health. Self-care for nurses starts with an awareness of personal needs and then finding ways to take care of them.

Resilience has been championed as a means of managing the stresses and strains of clinical practice and everyday life. Maintaining resilience can be as simple as remembering to take breaks, eat well and stay hydrated at work. We know that many staff overlook these things as they battle with heavy workloads and staff shortages, but failure to look after yourself can make workloads and staff shortages even worse if you end up having to take time off. It is important that we look after ourselves in order to look after others.

Activities: Brief outline answers

Activity 11.1   Reflection (page 172)

Steps you can take to look after yourself:

- Plan when you take your break, discuss with other nurses when they are going and make sure you can take turns to cover the other nurses' roles.
- Take a bottle of water with you and have this at the nurses' station; you can buy certain water bottles that indicate hourly how much you should be drinking.
- When you have a day off, prepare healthy meals so you can put them in the fridge or freeze them – use online websites to find ideas.
- Set a time or an alarm to be in bed so you can ensure you do get a good night's sleep.
- Take time to relax – run a warm bath in the evening or read a book to help focus your mind on other things.
- Get a diary and factor in time to see family or friends – the key is planning in advance.
- Walk part way to work or, if you prefer, take evening walks, runs or cycles. Visit the local sports centre and see if there are any gym classes or free outdoor events (e.g. local runs) that you can participate in around work.

Further reading

Brennan, EJ (2017) Towards Resilience and Well-Being in Nurses. *British Journal of Nursing*, 26(1): 43–7.

This paper suggests a number of methods to improve resilience.

Royal College of Nursing (RCN) (2015) *Stress and You: A Guide for Nursing Staff.* Available at: www.rcn.org.uk/professional-development/publications/pub-004967

This booklet provides advice on how you can reduce stress and manage your responses more effectively, as well as what to expect from your employer in terms of support.

Useful websites

www.mindful.org/meditation/mindfulness-getting-started/

This is a useful resource and introduction to the practice of mindfulness.

www.nhs.uk/live-well/eat-well/the-eatwell-guide/

Visit the NHS Eat Well Guide website for more information on achieving a balanced diet.

www.rcn.org.uk/healthy-workplace/healthy-workplaces

You can find more information about how to protect your resilience in the RCN's *Healthy Workplace, Healthy You* publications. This is a great resource.

www.sleepfoundation.org

The Sleep Foundation is dedicated to improving health and well-being through sleep education and advocacy.

www.sleepstation.org.uk/articles/

Sleepstation provides articles and research about sleep and insomnia.

https://thesleepcharity.org.uk/information-support/adults/sleep-hygiene/

The Sleep Charity's aim is to help you get a better night's sleep.

Chapter 12 Future trends: challenges and opportunities in health promotion

Chapter aims

After reading this chapter, you will be able to:

- begin to develop an understanding of **globalisation** and its influence on health and well-being;
- consider the influence of politics that impact on health and well-being;
- explore how an understanding of health and well-being needs across the lifespan is influencing the future of service provision;
- identify how service delivery is changing, as well as the importance of sustainable **integrated care systems** to the future of healthcare provision.

> ## Case study: Dominique
>
> Dominique is 84 and a retired nurse. She is living in a nursing home and is talking to her grandson, who has just started his nurse training.
>
> *You know, when I started nursing back in the sixties, it was nothing like it is now. So much changed during my career. People were old at 60, and it wasn't unusual to hear of people dying well before they were 70. Most of my patients were white and British in the early days, so they used to think it strange to have a black nurse looking after them. That changed when more people from other countries moved to the UK to work.*
>
> *Over time, the focus in our work changed too. Of course, we always cared for people, you can't get away from that, but we did it with more and more machines, different medicines and new techniques. Nurses started to have a bigger voice too. Just getting a degree means you have more respect than I did with my enrolled nurse registration. I expect you will see that when you get out from university and into the clinical areas. There was so much improvement in what we knew about diseases and keeping healthy that we started talking to people more and more about managing their health when they were at home.*
>
> *I often look around at the other residents here and realise we are all a lot older than most of the patients back in my day. But we all have health needs that sometimes make it really hard being old. At least we have the NHS and the social care system. Mind you, with the state of politics nowadays, I do worry. I hope the NHS keeps going as I don't think people will be able to afford healthcare if they have to pay for everything. That would be such a backward step.*

Introduction

There has been a significant change in the knowledge and practice of nursing over the past century. This has been influenced by changes in the provision of health services in the UK, the advancements in knowledge of health conditions and the understanding of the impact of lifestyle and wider determinants of health on the health and well-being of people.

The case study above reflects that change is always happening. As nurses, we are not passengers to that change, but key drivers of change. We have the opportunity to work with people and multi-professional colleagues to influence, lead and manage developments in healthcare provision. Therefore, we must all have an awareness of the wider influences that are impacting on the population and the health and social care services in which we work. Being cognisant of significant influences on health and well-being will enable effective developments in health promotion for future care delivery.

This chapter brings the book to a conclusion. We will explore the current influences on health and well-being nationally and globally. This will include the impact of globalisation on the movement of people, as well as how being culturally competent is essential to the provision of health promotion in a diverse society. We will consider the political landscape and the potential influence on individual and population health. We will also consider some of the current elements impacting the health and well-being of sectors of the population across the lifespan, as well as the importance of providing responsive, person-centred care. Finally, we will address the impact and opportunities in developments in healthcare delivery systems, as well as how these have the potential to advance the approaches to improve population health.

Globalisation

We begin this chapter by briefly considering the concept of globalisation. Pre-pandemic, globalisation was a key international strategy, impacting on the trade relationships between countries, how they interacted on the political stage and how countries managed and addressed key social, health and economic issues that impacted on global and national communities (Bradbury-Jones and Clark, 2017). It also encouraged migration of skilled workers, building international links in many areas including research, science and health. Globalisation aimed to enable transformative commitments to address health and well-being, reducing inequalities within and across populations. An example is the UN Sustainable Development Goals (SDGs) (UN, 2015), an international commitment that addresses 17 key areas which impact on the health and well-being of populations, including poverty, education and climate change. We encourage you to explore the UN SDGs website as this commitment is influential in both UK and international policy developments (see the useful websites section at the end of the chapter).

Globalisation and health service delivery

Globalisation enabled the movement of people, products and services across borders. This has benefited the NHS in recent years with the migration of skilled healthcare workers to the UK to address staffing issues. However, policies to make movement of people across borders easier also increased the movement of documented and undocumented people across borders who may require healthcare services. In particular, the migration of people who are unvaccinated increases the transmission of communicable diseases and the risk of localised disease outbreaks such as tuberculosis or measles. Some people may also arrive in the UK having not had the opportunity to access healthcare in their home countries, and therefore have untreated existing physical or mental health needs. They are likely to need additional support to access NHS services due to cultural and language barriers.

Increasing diversity in the UK population means it is essential that culturally competent approaches meet the social, linguistic and cultural needs of people. Application of a homogenous approach to the provision of services in a culturally and ethnically diverse population results in a non-inclusive, culturally insensitive approach to service provision and delivery, which further alienates and disempowers those who potentially need greater support. Communication, collaboration and truly understanding the needs of a particular community are essential in developing services and resources, empowering people and meeting health outcomes (CQC, 2022). While provision of care to a multi-cultural population may present a challenge to service delivery, it is one that we must embrace to maintain our core professional values on the provision of person-centred care. You may become involved, or indeed lead, on the essential work with communities and within the organisations where you work to ensure that culturally accessible services are available. This may include designing brand new services or even a radical review of current health promotion approaches to ensure resources and practitioner knowledge reflect the cultural needs of people.

National political influences

The COVID-19 pandemic has had significant impacts on the progress of globalisation policies nationally and internationally. Lagarde (2021) asserts that pre-pandemic globalisation strategies meant that countries were susceptible to the impact of global shocks. Although during the pandemic there was a global effort in public health strategies to share knowledge, science and resources to combat the virus, around the world countries implemented restrictions to protect their populations that impacted on globalisation policies. National interests increased, trade and services were limited, leading to restrictions in availability of some goods and services, and some people lost their main source of income due to businesses being closed. In the UK, Marmot et al. (2020) articulate the significance of UK pandemic policies on people, including the increase in deprivation, poverty and associated negative impacts on health and well-being.

As nurses we do not need to be 'experts' on global issues, but the pandemic has brought into stark focus that it is necessary for us to have an awareness of both global and national issues that ultimately have an influence on people's health and well-being. You will be at the forefront of person-centred care that is responsive to people's needs, so it is important that you use this knowledge to innovate in your nursing practice and to promote health and well-being in the communities where you work.

Being cognisant of the political policies and agendas is important in nursing practice. Political decisions not only impact on the health and well-being of people we provide services to, but also on our profession in terms of working conditions, staffing and ongoing development of high-quality evidence-based practice through research and collaboration. At the end of this chapter, we provide you with some links to key publications which will help you to develop an understanding of these issues.

Political instability within a country can have implications for the population. In 2016, the UK population voted in a referendum to leave the EU ('Brexit'). This resulted in repercussions for the dynamics of UK politics and the relationship with the EU (UK in a Changing Europe, 2019). Many people have been concerned about the implications of Brexit on several topics, including immigration, maintaining the NHS in the public domain and access to pharmaceutical products (Baird and McKenna, 2019).

In Activity 12.1, you will consider how the political landscape in the UK has influenced healthcare provision.

> ## Activity 12.1   Critical thinking and reflection
>
> Critically reflect on the following: Since the 2016 referendum, how have the UK Government developed the UK's position globally? What trade deals have been developed that increase opportunities for employment, movement of goods and services and support the movement of skilled workers to the UK? What are the opportunities for collaborations between clinical researchers internationally? What have been the negative impacts of loss of traditional trade partners or research collaborations? How has the UK's political position with the EU impacted on the NHS, the provision of health and social care services, and the availability of key resources such as healthcare staff and medicines? What has been the response of healthcare organisations, unions, staff and service users?
>
> *This is a reflective activity; therefore, there is no outline answer at the end of the chapter.*

In terms of impacts on people, communities and the population, it is helpful to consider the wider determinants of health when you reflect on the above activity. Hopefully you will be able to come to a critical understanding of the impact of the political landscape in the UK on the population, and whether the health and well-being of the population, and the provision of health services, have been adversely or positively impacted by Brexit. Large companies may withdraw their production in UK-based factories or increase their investment following better trade deals, impacting on employment and unemployment rates. Families may become more financially stable or need to rely on social welfare payments (benefits). The impact on the NHS may become significant with increased investment versus privatisation. The availability of international healthcare staff may decrease as they return to their home countries, leaving posts vacant and increasing the pressures on an already stretched healthcare workforce. Availability of medicines and medical equipment may become restricted, impacting on millions of people, including those with long-term health needs. Whatever the consequences, it is increasingly important that we have a political awareness to advocate for our profession, as well as the needs of the health service and the population. Subsequently, our active engagement with current political issues is vitally important.

Future population needs across the lifespan

There are many topics which we could focus on in this section. However, we have focused on two elements which are important, regardless of the field of nursing you are studying. The first topic is the rising awareness of poor mental health within people across the lifespan. Wherever you work you will engage with people who have mental health needs. You will be an integral part of providing services that ensure mental health needs of people are met. Healthcare provision needs to not only address the needs of people with diagnosed mental health conditions to support and empower them to manage their physical and mental health needs, but also services need to be focused to support people who do not have a diagnosed mental health condition to maintain or develop their mental well-being.

The UK's Office for Health Improvement and Disparities (2022d) reports that for some people the pandemic has had a negative impact on their mental health. The data suggests there are a range of factors that may have resulted in poorer mental health. Negative influences on mental health include lockdowns, the psychological impact of being seriously ill with the virus, caring for people who have been ill and/or died and the isolation felt especially by those who had been shielding. With all education being remotely delivered, people being furloughed, social events being cancelled and restrictions on travel and contact with family and friends, people of all ages reported feeling isolated, lonely and depressed.

The mental health sector is seeing an increase in use of services, and a rise in diagnoses of eating disorders, depression and post-traumatic stress disorder. Whether you are a children and young people's nurse, an adult nurse or a learning disability nurse, collaboration with mental health nurses and other mental health professionals will enable you to develop an understanding of mental health needs and disorders to effectively provide appropriate and supportive healthcare.

The second topic which has importance for all fields of nursing is the morbidity and mortality of people living with learning disabilities and autism. Across their lifespan they will access acute and community services and so it is a sobering fact for all healthcare professionals to acknowledge that for many people living with a learning disability, access to healthcare and person-centred treatment while using healthcare services requires significant improvement. It has been acknowledged that 'diagnostic overshadowing' (assuming the presenting behaviour is related to the disability rather than the physical health need) is a significant influence on people receiving inadequate treatment, particularly when people with learning disabilities require inpatient acute care. Efforts to reduce unconscious bias and provide person-centred, effective and specialised care is a target in the NHS Long Term Plan (NHS England, 2019a). The Learning Disability Mortality Review (LeDeR) Programme (2019) indicates a significant disparity between age of death for those with a learning disability and the general population. For people living with learning disabilities, there is an increased potential for physical and mental health comorbidities; therefore, focused health promotion activities, adapted to meet their needs is essential and necessary.

Changes in health service delivery

Healthcare provision has changed over several decades, reflecting a shift from acute to community services (HEE, 2017). Developing sustainable services requires collaboration and integration between systems (both physical provision of services and integrated IT systems), as well as services to deliver health and social care to target specific populations. You will be working within a healthcare service which will have integrated healthcare at the heart of effective service provision so it is important that you understand how these changes will impact your practice and service delivery.

The NHS

Buck et al. (2018) suggest that the NHS should be considered as a wider determinant of health as the provision of free healthcare mitigates income inequalities in the population. Therefore, as an asset, the NHS needs to be responsive to the delivery of healthcare locally and nationally to drive forward change for future population health.

The NHS Long Term Plan acknowledged the changing dynamics in healthcare systems, population health needs and the importance of effective and responsive service delivery (NHS England, 2019a). It highlighted the transformation of the way people use services, as well as the importance of developing services that are responsive to people's needs and engage them in taking responsibility for their health and well-being.

With an increasing community focus, there is the commitment to the development of primary care networks (e.g. GP practices, community teams), physical and Mental Health Services and the integration of health and social care services as integral to the Integrated Care Systems approach (NHS England, 2019b). In 2022 Integrated Care Systems became statutory bodies, with multiple health, social care and allied agencies working together to deliver health and social care within localities in the UK (Health and Care Act 2022). Therefore, it is essential that we understand how these systems will influence how we provide care, working with people and the multi-agency team.

As nurses, we will continue to provide care that is responsive to the changing needs of the populations and health systems within which we work. Developing your understanding of the various elements that impact on the health and well-being of people, families, communities and populations, both globally and nationally, is not only essential in effective care delivery, but also in the improvement of sustainable health service development.

Identifying the needs of targeted groups of people requires an overall awareness of population health trends, a focused awareness of the needs of people in your local geographical area and a clear understanding of the needs and experiences of the particular people with whom you are working closely. Essential to our practice is working closely within interdisciplinary and multi-professional teams and local services, as well as closely collaborating with people, families and communities to develop sustainable innovations in practice.

Chapter summary

This chapter has explored the challenges and opportunities in promoting health and well-being within populations. We have briefly considered the influence of globalisation and its impact on healthcare. We have also explored how the political landscape can influence population and global policies that impact on health and well-being. Finally, we identified healthcare developments that impact on people across the lifespan, before focusing on current and future implications of changes to health service delivery.

Useful websites

www.cqc.org.uk/publications/major-report/state-care

To understand the issues impacting on the 'State of Care' in the UK, read this 2022 publication from the CQC.

www.england.nhs.uk/integratedcare/integrated-care-systems

For further information about Integrated Care Systems in the UK.

www.globalgoals.org

For further information about the UN Sustainable Development Goals.

www.kingsfund.org.uk/publications/health-and-care-act-key-questions

To support your understanding of the importance of the Health and Care Act 2022, the King's Fund has provided a long-read article, *The Health and Care Act: Six Key Questions.*

Glossary of key terms

6Cs   Nurses operate on six core values, commonly known as the 6Cs. These are care, compassion, competence, communication, courage and commitment.

arthroscopy   A type of keyhole surgery used to diagnose and treat problems with joints.

autonomy   The right of patients to make decisions about their care, health and well-being without their nurse or other healthcare professional trying to influence the decision. Patient autonomy does allow for healthcare providers to educate the patient, but does not allow the healthcare provider to make the decision for the patient.

COPD   A lung disease known as Chronic Obstructive Pulmonary Disease.

coping strategies   The specific behavioural and psychological efforts utilised by people to manage stressful life events.

country of origin   The country from which a person originally came.

data sets   A collection of sets of statistical information that have been categorised.

digital technology   Essentially, the breakdown of messages, signals or forms of communication between the creating device and the receiving device through the use of a string of information known as binary code.

e-government   The use of information and communication technologies (ICTs) to improve the activities of public sector organisations.

evaluation framework   Provides an overall framework for evaluations across different programmes or different evaluations of a single programme. It sometimes includes an overall programme theory/logic model and principles to guide the planning, management and conduct of evaluations.

evidence-based practice   Within nursing, achieved by developing and supporting patient-centred approaches to care using the most current evidence available.

globalisation   The process of the increasing interconnectedness between countries, involving political, economic, health and social issues.

Fitbit   A wearable computing device. It is a fitness band, worn on a person's wrist, and is designed to track physical activity. Fitbit devices are designed to track important health and activity markers, including heart rate, quality of sleep and the number of steps walked.

Health behaviours   The modifiable behaviours and lifestyle choices that impact on an individual's health and well-being.

health literacy   The ability and capacity for people to access, process and understand health information to make decisions about their health.

herd immunity   When the majority of the population is immunised, this limits the transition of a disease, providing protection to those who are unable to be immunised.

holistically   The way in which the nurse treats the whole person, taking into account mental and social factors, rather than just the symptoms of a disease.

integrated care systems   Partnerships with local statutory and related services to manage resources and meet NHS standards to improve the health of local populations.

intranet   A private enterprise network designed to support an organisation's employees to communicate, collaborate and perform their roles. It serves a broad range of purposes and uses, but at its core an intranet is there to help employees.

life course   The roles and processes that people engage in throughout their lives.

lifestyle   The way in which a person lives. Lifestyle is the interests, opinions, behaviours and behavioural orientations of an individual, group or culture.

marginalised   The relegation of a person or social group to a lowly position in society.

minority group   Membership is typically based on differences in observable characteristics or practices, such as ethnicity (ethnic minority), race (racial minority), religion (religious minority), sexual orientation (sexual minority), disability, or gender identity.

mobile application interface   The graphical and usually touch-sensitive display on a mobile device, such as a smartphone or tablet, that allows the user to interact with the device's apps, features, content and functions.

motivational interviewing   A counselling method that helps people resolve ambivalent feelings and insecurities to find the internal motivation they need to change their behaviour. It is a practical, empathetic and short-term process that takes into consideration how difficult it is to make life changes.

personal bias   We all hold our own subjective world views and are influenced and shaped by our experiences, beliefs, values, education, family, friends, peers and others. Being aware of one's biases is vital to both personal well-being and professional success.

poverty   People living in poverty do not have enough material or financial means to meet their needs.

public health surveillance   The ongoing collection and analysis of health-related data that are used to plan, implement and evaluate public health approaches.

revalidation   The process that all nurses and midwives in the UK and nursing associates in England need to follow to maintain their registration with the NMC.

SARS-CoV-2   The official name of the causative virus commonly known as COVID-19.

social capital   The ability of members of a society to engage in effective networks and relationships to improve the effective functioning of the society.

social ecological model   A model that enables consideration of the multiple factors that influence people's lifestyles and behaviours.

stereotype   A simplified assumption about a group based on prior experiences or beliefs. Stereotypes can be positive (e.g. 'women are warm and nurturing') or negative (e.g. 'teenagers are lazy').

Troubled Families Programme   A programme of targeted intervention for families with multiple problems, including crime, antisocial behaviour, truancy, unemployment, mental health problems and domestic abuse.

References

Age UK (2014) *Fit as a Fiddle: Engaging Faith and BME Communities in Activities and Wellbeing*. London: Age UK.

Atkinson, J (2000) *European Foundation for the Improvement of Living and Working Conditions: Employment Options and Labour Market Participation*. Luxembourg: Office for Official Publications of the European Communities.

Baird, B and McKenna, H (2019) *Brexit: The Implications for Health and Social Care*. Available at: www.kingsfund.org.uk/publications/articles/brexit-implications-health-social-care

Bajwa, M (2014) Emerging 21st Century Medical Technologies. *Pakistan Journal of Medical Sciences*, 30(3): 649–55.

Bandura, A (1997) *Self-Efficacy: The Exercise of Control*. New York: W.H. Freeman.

Bennett, BL, Goldstein, CM, Gathright, EC, Hughes, JW and Latnera, JD (2017) Internal Health Locus of Control Predicts Willingness to Track Health Behaviours Online and with Smartphone Applications. *Psychology, Health and Medicine*, 22(10): 1224–9.

Berg, L, Skott, C and Danielson, E (2007) Caring Relationship in a Context: Fieldwork in a Medical Ward. *International Journal of Nursing Practice*, 13(2): 100–6.

Better Health (2021) *About and Contact: What Is Better Health?* Available at: https://www.nhs.uk/healthier-families/about-and-contact/

Better Health (2022) *Quit Smoking*. Available at: https://www.nhs.uk/better-health/quit-smoking/

Better Health-Healthier Families (2022) *Easy Ways To Eat Well And Move More*. Available at: https://www.nhs.uk/healthier-families/

Bhat, SA, Darzi, MA and Hakim, IA (2019) Understanding Social Marketing and Well-Being: A Review of Selective Databases. *Vikalpa*, 44(2): 1–13.

Bottery, S, Ward, D and Fenney, D (2019) *Social Care 360*. Available at: www.kingsfund.org.uk/publications/social-care-360

Bradbury-Jones, C and Clark, M (2017) Globalisation and Global Health: Issues for Nursing. *Nursing Standard*, 31(39): 54–63.

Bronfenbrenner, U (2005) *Making Human Beings Human: Bioecological Perspectives on Human Development*. Thousand Oaks, CA: SAGE.

Buchvold, HV, Pallesen, S, Nicolas, MF and Bjorvatn, B (2015) Associations Between Night Work and BMI, Alcohol, Smoking, Caffeine and Exercise: A Cross-Sectional Study. *BMC Public Health*, 15: 1112.

Buck, D and Wenzel, L (2018) *Communities and Health*. Available at: www.kingsfund.org.uk/publications/communities-and-health

Buck, D, Baylis, A, Dougall, D and Robertson, R (2018) *A Vision for Population Health: Towards a Healthier Future.* Available at: www.kingsfund.org.uk/publications/vision-population-health

Calderón-Larrañaga S, Greenhalgh T, Finer S and Clinch M (2022) What Does the Literature Mean by Social Prescribing? A Critical Review Using Discourse Analysis. *Sociology of Health and Illness.* 2022, 1–21. Available at: https://onlinelibrary.wiley.com/doi/10.1111/1467-9566.13468

Care Act (2014). Available at: https://www.legislation.gov.uk/ukpga/2014/23/contents/enacted

Care Quality Commission (CQC) (2022) *Culturally appropriate care.* Available at: https://www.cqc.org.uk/guidance-providers/adult-social-care/culturally-appropriate-care

Centers for Disease Control and Prevention (CDC) (2011) *Introduction to Programme Evaluation for Public Health Programmes: A Self-Study Guide.* Atlanta, GA: US Department of Health and Human Services.

Centers for Disease Control and Prevention (2022) *Section 4: Program Evaluation in Six Steps.* https://www.cdc.gov/visionhealth/programs/vision-health-toolkit/section-four/six-step-evaluation.html

Cherrill, L and Linsley, P (2017) The Use of Information and Communication Technologies in Mental Health Nursing. *British Journal of Mental Health Nursing,* 6(3): 118–22.

Chikhradze, N, Knecht, C and Metzing, S (2017) Young Carers: Growing Up With Chronic Illness in the Family – A Systematic Review 2007–2017. *Journal of Compassionate Health Care* 4(12). Available at: https:/jcompassionatehc.biomedcentral.com/track/pdf/10.1186/s40639-017-0041-3.pdf

Coggon, J and Adams J (2021) 'Let Them Choose Not to Eat Cake…': Public Health Ethics, Effectiveness and Equity in Government Obesity Strategy. *Future Healthcare Journal,* Vol 8 (No.1) 49–52. Available at: https://www.rcpjournals.org/content/futurehosp/8/1/49

Collins, B (2015) *Making Every Contact Count: Rapid Evidence Review.* Liverpool: University of Liverpool, Wirral Council Business and Public Health Intelligence Team.

Corace, KM, Stigley, JA, Hargadon, DP, Yu, D, MacDonald, TK and Fabrigar, LR (2016) Using Behaviour Change Frameworks to Improve Healthcare Worker Influenza Vaccination Rates: A Systematic Review. *Vaccine,* 34(28): 3235–42.

Cotton, R, Irwin, J, Wilkins, A and Young, C (2014) *The Future's Digital: Mental Health and Technology.* London: Mental Health Network.

Coughlin, SS (2008) How Many Principles for Public Health Ethics? *The Open Public Health Journal,* 1(1): 8–16.

Coughlin, SS and Stewart, J (2016) Use of Consumer Wearable Devices to Promote Physical Activity: A Review of Health Intervention Studies. *Journal of Environment and Health Studies,* 2(6): 1–6.

Coulter, A (2009) *Engaging Communities for Health Improvement: A Scoping Study for the Health Foundation.* London: Health Foundation.

Cross, T, Bazron, B, Dennis, K and Isaacs, M (1989) *Towards a Culturally Competent System of Care, Volume I.* Washington, DC: Georgetown University Child Development Center, CASSP Technical Assistance Center.

Dahlgren, G and Whitehead, M (1991) *Policies and Strategies to Promote Social Equity in Health.* Stockholm: Institute for Future Studies.

Davoodvand, S, Abbaszadeh, A and Ahmadi, F (2016) Patient Advocacy from the Clinical Nurses' Viewpoint: A Qualitative Study. *Journal of Medical Ethics and History of Medicine,* 9: 5.

Department for Business, Energy and Industrial Strategy (2022) *Annual Fuel Poverty Statistics in England, 2022* (2020 data). Available at: https://assets.publishing.service. gov.uk/government/uploads/system/uploads/attachment_data/file/1056842/fuel-poverty-factsheet-2020.pdf

Department for Work and Pensions (DWP) (2020) *Family Resources Survey 2018/2019.* Available at: https://assets.publishing.service.gov.uk/government/uploads/system/uploads/attachment_data/file/874507/family-resources-survey-2018-19.pdf

Department of Health (DH) (1998) *Independent Inquiry into Inequalities in Health.* London: The Stationery Office.

Department of Health (DH) (2010) *Healthy Lives, Healthy People: Our Strategy for Public Health in England.* London: DH.

Department of Health (DH) (2011) *The New Public Health System: Summary.* London: DH.

Department of Health (DH) (2012) *Long Term Conditions Compendium of Information,* 3rd edition. London: DH.

Department of Health (DH) (2013) *The NHS Outcomes Framework 2014/15.* London: DH.

Department of Health and Social Care (DHSC) (2018) *Prevention Is Better Than Cure: Our Vision to Help You Live Well for Longer.* London: DHSC.

Department of Health and Social Care (DHSC) (2019) *UK Chief Medical Officers' Physical Activity Guidelines.* London: DHSC.

Department of Health and Social Security (DHSS) (1980) *Inequalities in Health: Report of a Research Working Group.* London: DHSS.

Dewhirst, VS (2015) *Wessex Making Every Contact Count: Evaluation Report.* Independent report from the Academic Unit of Primary Care and Population Sciences, University of Southampton, commissioned by the Wessex School of Public Health, Health Education Wessex (HEW), to evaluate the Wessex MECC approach.

Digital Health and Care Institute (DHI) (2019) *What Is Digital Health and Care?* Available at: https://www.legislation.gov.uk/ukpga/2014/23/contents/enacted

Draeger, E, Bedford, HE and Elliman, DAC (2019) Should Measles Vaccination be Compulsory? *British Medical Journal,* 365: 12359. Available at: https://doi.org/10.1136/bmj.l2359

Edwards, M, Carter, A, Hay, L and Graham, K (2018) *Health Coaching: Innovation and Adoption Stories of Impact from NHS Organisations.* Available at: https://www.betterconversation.co.uk/images/IES%20Report%20530_Organisational%20stories%20of%20impact%20from%20health%20coaching.pdf

Equality Act (2010) Available at: www.legislation.gov.uk/ukpga/2010/15/contents

Equality and Human Rights Commission (EHRC) (2016) *Healing a Divided Britain: The Need for a Comprehensive Race Equality Strategy.* London: EHRC.

European Commission (EC) (2018) *Market Study on Telemedicine.* Brussels: EC.

Eysenbach, G (2001) What is eHealth? *Journal of Medical Internet Research,* 3(2): e20.

Feist, HR, Parker, K and Graeme, H (2012) Older and Online: Enhancing Social Connections in Australian Rural Places. *The Journal of Community Informatics,* 8(1). Available at: https://openjournals.uwaterloo.ca/index.php/JoCI/article/view/3068/3977

Finnis, A, Khan, H, Ejbye, J, Wood, S and Redding, D (2016) *Realising the Value: Ten Key Steps to Put People and Communities at the Heart of Health and Wellbeing.* Available at: www.nesta.org.uk/report/realising-the-value-ten-actions-to-put-people-and-communities-at-the-heart-of-health-and-wellbeing/

Fitzpatrick, L (2018) The Importance of Communication and Professional Values Relating to Nursing Practice. *Links to Health and Social Care,* 3(1): 27–40.

Forbes, AE, Schutzer-Weissmann, J, Menassa, DA and Wilson, MH (2017) Head Injury Patterns in Helmeted and Non-Helmeted Cyclists. *PLOS One,* 12(9): e0185367.

Foster, HME, Celis-Morales, CA, Nicholl, BI, Petermann-Rocha, F, Pell, JP and Gill, JMR (2018) The Effect of Socioeconomic Deprivation on the Association Between an Extended Measurement of Unhealthy Lifestyle Factors and Health Outcomes: A Prospective Analysis of the UK Biobank Cohort. *The Lancet Public Health,* 3(12): e576–e585.

Glanz, K, Rimer, BK and Lewis, FM (2002) *Health Behaviour and Health Education: Theory, Research and Practice.* San Francisco, CA: Wiley & Sons.

Godlee, F, Smith, J and Marcovitch, H (2011) Wakefield's Article Linking MMR Vaccine and Autism was Fraudulent. *British Medical Journal,* 342: c7452.

Grier, S and Bryant, CA (2005) Social Marketing in Public Health. *Annual Review of Public Health,* 26(1): 319–39.

Gruman, JA, Schneider, FW and Coutts, LM (eds) (2016). *Applied Social Psychology: Understanding and Addressing Social and Practical Problems.* ProQuest Ebook Central https://ebookcentral.proquest.com

Haque, Z, Becares, L & Treloar, N (2020) Over-Exposed and Under-Protected – The Devastating Impact of COVID-19 on Black and Minority Ethnic Communities in Great Britain. Runnymede Trust, London.

Harding, M and Jarvis, S (2019) *Audit and Audit Cycle.* Available at: https://patient.info/doctor/audit-and-audit-cycle

Health and Care Act (2022) Available at: https://www.legislation.gov.uk/ukpga/2022/31/contents/enacted

Health Education England (HEE) (2017) *Health Literacy 'How To' Guide.* Available at: https://library.nhs.uk/wp-content/uploads/sites/4/2020/08/Health-literacy-how-to-guide.pdf

Health Education England (HEE) (2019a) *Integrated Care.* Available at: www.hee.nhs.uk/our-work/integrated-care

Health Education England (HEE) (2019b) *NHS Staff and Learners' Mental Wellbeing Commission.* Available at: https://www.hee.nhs.uk/sites/default/files/documents/NHS%20%28HEE%29%20-%20Mental%20Wellbeing%20Commission%20Report.pdf?dm_i=21A8,64W3H,ITDDXX,O4KCX,1

Health Foundation (2015) *Evaluation: What to Consider – Commonly Asked Questions about How to Approach Evaluation of Quality Improvement in Health Care.* London: Health Foundation.

Heart Foundation (2019) *Fruit, Vegetables and Wholegrains.* Available at: www.heartfoundation. org.au/healthy-eating/food-and-nutrition/fruit-vegetables-and-wholegrains

Hibbard, J and Gilburt, H (2014) *Supporting People to Manage Their Health: An Introduction to Patient Activation.* Available at: www.kingsfund.org.uk/sites/default/files/field/field_ publication_file/supporting-people-manage-health-patient-activation-may14.pdf

HM Government (2018a) *A Connected Society: A Strategy for Tackling Loneliness – Laying the Foundations for Change.* London: HM Government.

HM Government (2018b) *Population of England and Wales.* Available at: www.ethnicity-facts-figures.service.gov.uk/uk-population-by-ethnicity/national-and-regional-populations/ population-of-england-and-wales/latest

HM Government (2018c) *Working Together to Safeguard Children: A Guide to Inter-Agency Working to Safeguard and Promote the Welfare of Children.* Available at: https://assets. publishing.service.gov.uk/government/uploads/system/uploads/attachment_data/ file/942454/Working_together_to_safeguard_children_inter_agency_guidance.pdf

HM Government (2019) *List of Ethnic Groups.* Available at: www.ethnicity-facts-figures. service.gov.uk/ethnic-groups

Holland, K and Hogg, C (2010) *Cultural Awareness in Nursing and Health Care: An Introductory Text,* 2nd edition. London: Routledge.

Holmes, J (2021) Tackling Obesity: The Role of the NHS in a Whole-System Approach. Available at: https://www.kingsfund.org.uk/sites/default/files/2021-07/Tackling%20 obesity.pdf

Homelessness Act (2002). Available at: www.legislation.gov.uk/ukpga/2002/7/contents

Hornby-Turner, YC, Peel, NM and Hubbard, RE (2017) Health Assets in Older Age: A Systematic Review. *British Medical Journal Open,* 7(5): 1–13.

Housing Act (1996). Available at: www.legislation.gov.uk/ukpga/1996/52/contents

Housing (Homeless Persons) Act (1977). Available at: https://www.legislation.gov.uk/ ukpga/1977/48/contents/enacted

Hutchinson, J and Smith, AD (1996) Introduction, in Hutchinson, J and Smith, AD (eds), *Ethnicity.* Oxford: Oxford University Press.

International Rescue Committee (IRC) (2018) *Migrants, Asylum Seekers, Refugees and Immigrants: What's the Difference?* Available at: www.rescue.org/article/migrants-asylum-seekers-refugees-and-immigrants-whats-difference

James, N (2013) The Formal Support Experiences of Family Carers of People with an Intellectual Disability Who Also Display Challenging Behaviour and/or Mental Health Issues: What Do Carers Say? *Journal of Intellectual Disabilities,* 17(1): 6–23.

Jeffery, D (2016) Empathy, Sympathy and Compassion in Healthcare. Is There a Problem? Is There a Difference? Does it Matter? *Journal of the Royal Society of Medicine,* 109(12): 446–52.

Jordan, SE, Hovet, SE, Chun-Hai, I, Liang, H, Fu, K-W and Tszz Ho Tse, Z (2018) Using Twitter for Public Health Surveillance from Monitoring and Prediction to Public Response. *Data,* 4: 6.

Joseph Rowntree Foundation (2022) *UK Poverty 2022: The Essential Guide to Understanding Poverty in the UK*. York: Joseph Rowntree Foundation. Available at: https://www.jrf.org.uk/report/uk-poverty-2022

King's Fund (2018a) *A Vision for Population Health: Towards a Healthier Future*. London: King's Fund.

King's Fund (2018b) *Transformational Change in Health and Care: Reports from the Field*. London: King's Fund.

King's Fund (2022) *The Health and Care Act: Six Key Questions*. Available at: https://www.kingsfund.org.uk/publications/health-and-care-act-key-questions

Lagarde, C (2021) *Globalisation After the Pandemic* (speech). 2021 Per Jacobsson Lecture by Christine Lagarde, President of the ECB, at the IMF Annual Meetings. Available at: https://www.ecb.europa.eu/press/key/date/2021/html/ecb.sp211016~25550329d5.en.html

Lawrence, W, Black, C, Tinati, T, Cradock, S, Begum, R and Jarman, M (2014) 'Making Every Contact Count': Evaluation of the Impact of an Intervention to Train Health and Social Care Practitioners in Skills to Support Health Behaviour Change. *Journal of Health Psychology*, 21(2): 138–51.

Lazarus, RS and Folkman, S (1984) *Stress, Appraisal and Coping*. New York: Springer.

Learning Disability Mortality Review (LeDeR) Programme (2019) *Annual Report 2018*. Available at: www.hqip.org.uk/wp-content/uploads/2019/05/LeDeR-Annual-Report-Final-21-May-2019.pdf

Lee, E and Roberts, LJ (2018) Between Individual and Family Coping: A Decade of Theory and Research on Couples Coping With Health-Related Stress. *Journal of Family Theory and Review*, 10(1): 141–64.

Lee, L, Patel, T, Costa, A, Bryce, E, Hillier, LM and Slonim, K (2017) Screening for Frailty in Primary Care: Accuracy of Gait Speed and Hand-Grip Strength. *Canadian Family Physician*, 63(1): e51–e57.

Lewin, K (1951) *Field Theory in Social Science*, Cartwright, D (ed.). New York: Harper.

Lindstrom, Prof. B (2020) *Salutogenesis: An Introduction*. Available at: https://www.local.gov.uk/case-studies/salutogenesis-introduction

Linsley, P and Kane, R (2022) *Evidence-Based Practice for Nurses and Allied Health Professionals* (5th edition). London: Sage.

Lobo, R, Petrich, M and Burns, SK (2014) Supporting Health Promotion Practitioners to Undertake Evaluation for Program Development. *BMC Public Health*, 15: 1315.

Lupton, D (2014) Health Promotion in the Digital Era: A Critical Commentary. *Health Promotion International*, 31(1): 174–83.

Lupton, D (2015) *Digital Sociology*. London: Routledge.

Lyons, EJ, Lewis, ZH, Mayrsohn, BG and Rowland, JL (2014) Behaviour Change Techniques Implemented in Electronic Lifestyle Activity Monitors: A Systematic Content Analysis. *Journal of Medical Internet Research*, 16(8): e192.

Maguire, D, Evans, H, Honeyman, M and Omojomolo, D (2018) *Digital Change in Health and Social Care*. London: King's Fund.

Majumder, S, Aghayi, E, Noferesti, M, Memarzadeh-Tehran, H, Mondal, T and Pang, Z (2017) Smart Homes for Elderly Healthcare: Recent Advances and Research Challenges. *Sensors*, 17(11): e2496.

Markus, HR (2006) Who Am I? Identity, Race and Ethnicity, in Markus, HR and Moya, P (eds), *Doing Race: 21 Essays for the 21st Century*. New York: Norton.

Marmot, M (2010) *Fair Society, Healthy Lives: The Marmot Review*. Available at: https://www.instituteofhealthequity.org/resources-reports/fair-society-healthy-lives-the-marmot-review

Marmot, M, Allen, J, Boyce, T, Goldblatt, P and Morrison, J (2018) *Health Equity In England: The Marmot Review 10 Years On*. Available at: https://health.org.uk/publications/reports/the-marmot-review-10-years-on

Marmot, M, Allen, J, Goldblatt, P, Herd, E and Herd, E (2020) *Build Back Fairer: The COVID-19 Marmot Review: The Pandemic, Socioeconomic and Health Inequalities in England: Executive Summary*. Available at: https://www.instituteofhealthequity.org/resources-reports/build-back-fairer-the-covid-19-marmot-review/build-back-fairer-the-covid-19-marmot-review-executive-summary.pdf

Marsh, P and Glendenning, R (2005) *The Primary Care Service Evaluation Toolkit*. Leeds: National Co-ordinating Centre for Research Capacity Development.

Mason, P and Butler, CC (2010) *Health Behaviour Change: A Guide for Practitioners*. London: Churchill Livingstone/Elsevier.

Matsumoto, D (1996) *Culture and Psychology*. Pacific Grove, CA: Brooks/Cole.

Matthys, J, Elwyn, G, Van Nuland, M, Van Maele, G, De Sutter, A and De Meyere, M (2009) Patients' Ideas, Concerns, and Expectations (ICE) in General Practice: Impact on Prescribing. *British Journal of General Practice*, 59(558): 29–36.

McFadden, A, Siebelt, L, Gavine, A, Atkin, K, Bell, K and Innes, N (2018) Gypsy, Roma and Traveller Access to and Engagement with Health Services: A Systematic Review. *European Journal of Public Health*, 28(1): 74–81.

Menefee, HK, Thompson, MJ, Guterbock, TM, Williams, IC and Valdez, RS (2016) Mechanisms of Communicating Health Information Through Facebook: Implications for Consumer Health Information Technology Design. *Journal of Medical Internet Research*, 18(8): e218.

Mental Health Foundation (2019) *Guide to Investing in Your Relationships*. London: Mental Health Foundation.

Migration Data Portal (2019) *Migration and Health*. Available at: https://migrationdata portal.org/themes/migration-and-health

Miskir, Y and Emishaw, S (2018) Determinants of Nursing Process Implementation in North East Ethiopia: Cross-Sectional Study. *Nursing Research and Practice*, 7940854.

National Health Service (NHS) (2019a) *Benefits of Exercise*. Available at: www.nhs.uk/live-well/exercise/exercise-health-benefits/

National Health Service (NHS) (2019b) *How to Get to Sleep: Sleep and Tiredness*. Available at: www.nhs.uk/live-well/sleep-and-tiredness/how-to-get-to-sleep/

National Health Service (NHS) (2019d) *Walking for Health*. Available at: www.nhs.uk/live-well/exercise/walking-for-health/

National Health Service (NHS) (2019e) *The Eat Well Guide*. Available at: www.nhs.uk/live-well/eat-well/

National Institute for Health and Care Excellence (NICE) (2007) *Behaviour Change: General Approaches – Public Health Guideline 6.* Available at: www.nice.org.uk/guidance/ph6/chapter/3-Recommendations

National Institute for Health and Care Excellence (NICE) (2014a) *Behaviour Change: Individual Approaches – Public Health Guideline 49.* Available at: www.nice.org.uk/guidance/ph49/chapter/1-Recommendations

National Institute for Health and Care Excellence (NICE) (2014b) *Obesity: Identification, Assessment and Management.* Available at: www.nice.org.uk/guidance/cg189/chapter/1-Recommendations

National Institute for Health and Care Excellence (NICE) (2017) *Community Engagement: Improving Health and Wellbeing: Quality Standard [QS148].* Available at: https://www.nice.org.uk/guidance/qs148/resources/community-engagement-improving-health-and-wellbeing-pdf-75545486227141

National Institute for Health and Care Excellence (NICE) (2019a) *Glossary: Health Promotion.* Available at: www.nice.org.uk/glossary?letter=h

National Institute for Health and Care Excellence (NICE) (2019b) *NICE Impact Mental Health.* Available at: www.nice.org.uk/Media/Default/About/what-we-do/Into-practice/measuring-uptake/NICEimpact-mental-health.pdf

National Voices (2014) *Supporting Self-Management.* Available at: www.nationalvoices.org.uk/sites/default/files/public/publications/supporting_self-management.pdf

Naylor, C, Das, P, Ross, S, Honeyman, M, Thompson, J and Gilburt, H (2016) *Bringing Together Physical and Mental Health: A New Frontier for Integrated Care.* London: King's Fund.

Naylor, C and Wellings, D (2019) *A Citizen-Led Approach to Health and Care: Lessons from the Wigan Deal.* Available at: https://www.kingsfund.org.uk/publications/wigan-deal

Nelson, A, de Normanville, C, Payne, K and Kelly, MP (2013) Making Every Contact Count: An Evaluation. *Public Health,* 127(7): 653–60.

Newport, C (2019) *Digital Minimalism: Choosing a Focused Life in a Noisy World.* New York: Portfolio.

NHS (2019) *NHS Health Check.* Available at: https://www.nhs.uk/conditions/nhs-health-check/

NHS Digital (2018a) *Health Survey for England: Summary of Key Findings.* Available at: http://healthsurvey.hscic.gov.uk/support-guidance/public-health/health-survey-for-england-2018/key-findings.aspx

NHS Digital (2021a) *National Child Measurement Programme.* Available at: https://digital.nhs.uk/services/national-child-measurement-programme/

NHS Digital (2021b) *National Child Measurement Programme, England 2020/21 School Year: Part 4, Deprivation.* Available at: https://digital.nhs.uk/data-and-information/publications/statistical/national-child-measurement-programme/2020-21-school-year/deprivation

NHS Digital Service Manual (2021) *Content Style Guide: Health Literacy.* Available online at: https://service-manual.nhs.uk/content/health-literacy

NHS England (2014) *Making Every Contact Count (MECC) Project Evaluation Examples.* Available at: www.england.nhs.uk/wp-content/uploads/2014/06/mecc-case-studies.pdf

NHS England (2016) *NHS Standard Contract 2017/19.* Available at: www.england.nhs.uk/nhs-standard-contract/17-18/

NHS England (2017) *Accessible Information: Implementation Guidance v1.1.* Available at: https://www.england.nhs.uk/wp-content/uploads/2017/08/implementation-guidance.pdf

NHS England (2019a) *The NHS Long Term Plan.* Available at: https://longtermplan.nhs.uk

NHS England (2019b) *Integrated Care Systems.* Available at: https://www.england.nhs.uk/publication/integrated-care-systems-guidance/

NHS Future Forum (2012) *NHS Future Forum Summary Report.* Available at: www.gov.uk/government/publications/nhs-future-forum-recommendations-to-government-second-phase

NHS Health Scotland (2019) *What Are Health Inequalities?* Available at: www.healthscotland.scot/health-inequalities/what-are-health-inequalities

NHS Inform (2019) *Five Steps to Mental Wellbeing.* Available at: https://www.nhsinform.scot/healthy-living/mental-wellbeing/five-steps-to-mental-wellbeing

NHS Institute for Innovation and Improvement (2005) *Improvement Leaders' Guide: Evaluating Improvement – General Improvement Skills.* Nottingham: NHS Institute for Innovation and Improvement.

NHS Midlands and East (2012) *An Implementation Guide and Toolkit for Making Every Contact Count: Using Every Opportunity to Achieve Health and Wellbeing.* East Midlands Health Trainer Hub and NHS Derbyshire County.

NHS Wales (2019) *Person Centred Care.* Available at: www.wales.nhs.uk/governance-emanual/person-centred-care

Nursing and Midwifery Council (NMC) (2018a) *Future Nurse: Standards of Proficiency for Registered Nurses.* Available at: www.nmc.org.uk/globalassets/sitedocuments/education-standards/future-nurse-proficiencies.pdf

Nursing and Midwifery Council (NMC) (2018b) *The Code: Professional Standards of Practice and Behaviour for Nurses, Midwives and Nursing Associates.* Available at: www.nmc.org.uk/code

Nursing and Midwifery Council (NMC) (2021) *Standards of Proficiency for Specialist Community Public Health Nursing* (Issue DRAFT January). Available at: https://www.nmc.org.uk/globalassets/sitedocuments/post-registration/final-documents/standards-of-proficiency-for-specialist-community-public-health-nursing-.pdf

Office for Health Improvement and Disparities (2022a) Guidance Childhood Obesity: Applying All Our Health. Available at: https://www.gov.uk/government/publications/childhood-obesity-applying-all-our-health/childhood-obesity-applying-all-our-health

Office for Health Improvement and Disparities (2022b) *Wider Determinants of Health: Statistical Commentary,* May 2022 update. Available at: https://www.gov.uk/government/statistics/wider-determinants-of-health-may-2022-update/wider-determinants-of-health-statistical-commentary-may-2022-update

Office for Health Improvement and Disparities (2022c) *Wider Determinants of Health.* Available at: https://fingertips.phe.org.uk/profile/wider-determinants

Office for Health Improvement and Disparities (2022d) *COVID-19 Mental Health and Wellbeing Surveillance: Report.* Available at: https://www.gov.uk/government/publications/covid-19-mental-health-and-wellbeing-surveillance-report

Office for National Statistics (2021) *Coronavirus and Vaccine Hesitancy, Great Britain: 9 August 2021.* Available at: https://www.ons.gov.uk/peoplepopulationandcommunity/healthandsocialcare/healthandwell-being/bulletins/coronavirusandvaccinehesitancygreatbritain/9august2021

O'Mara-Eves, A, Brunton, G, McDaid, D, Oliver, S, Kavanagh, J and Jamal, F (2013) Community Engagement to Reduce Inequalities in Health: A Systematic Review, Meta-Analysis and Economic Analysis. *Public Health Research,* 1(4): 548.

Ossebaard, HC and van Gemert-Pijnen, L (2016) eHealth and Quality in Health Care: Implementation Time. *International Journal for Quality in Health Care,* 28(3): 415–19.

Parsons, T (1951) *The Social System.* Glencoe, IL: The Free Press.

Patel, MS, Asch, DA and Volpp, KG (2015) Wearable Devices as Facilitators, not Drivers, of Health Behaviour Change. *Journal of the American Medical Association,* 313(5): 459–60.

Patton, MQ (2018) Evaluation Science. *American Journal of Evaluation,* 39(2): 183–200.

Prochaska, JO and DiClemente, CC (1983) Stages and Processes of Self-Change of Smoking: Toward an Integrative Model of Change. *Journal of Consulting and Clinical Psychology,* 51(3): 390–5.

Public Health England (PHE) (2016) *Making Every Contact Count (MECC): Consensus Statement.* Available at: https://assets.publishing.service.gov.uk/government/uploads/system/uploads/attachment_data/file/769486/Making_Every_Contact_Count_Consensus_Statement.pdf

Public Health England (PHE) (2017) *Health Profile for England: 2017. Chapter 5: Inequality in Health.* Available at: www.gov.uk/government/publications/health-profile-for-england

Public Health England (PHE) (2018a) *Guidance: Health Matters – Preventing Type 2 Diabetes.* Available at: www.gov.uk/government/publications/health-matters-preventing-type-2-diabetes/health-matters-preventing-type-2-diabetes

Public Health England (2018b) *Guidance: Health Matters: Community-Centred Approaches for Health and Wellbeing.* https://www.gov.uk/government/publications/health-matters-health-and-wellbeing-community-centred-approaches/health-matters-community-centred-approaches-for-health-and-wellbeing

Public Health England (PHE) (2019a) *National Child Measurement Programme: A Conversation Framework for Talking to Parents.* Available at: https://assets.publishing.service.gov.uk/government/uploads/system/uploads/attachment_data/file/788813/NCMP_Conversation_framework_for_talking_to_parents.pdf

Public Health England (PHE) (2019b) *Guidance: Health Matters: Prevention – A Life Course Approach.* Available at: www.gov.uk/government/publications/health-matters-life-course-approach-to-prevention/health-matters-prevention-a-life-course-approach

Public Health England (PHE) (2019c) *UK Measles and Rubella Elimination Strategy 2019.* Available at: https://assets.publishing.service.gov.uk/government/uploads/system/uploads/attachment_data/file/769970/UK_measles_and_rubella_elimination_strategy.pdf

Public Health England (PHE) (2020a) *Achieving Behaviour Change: A Guide for National Government.* Available at: https://assets.publishing.service.gov.uk/government/uploads/system/uploads/attachment_data/file/933328/UFG_National_Guide_v04.00__1___1_.pdf

Public Health England (PHE) (2020b) *Analysis of the Relationship Between Pre-existing Health Conditions, Ethnicity and COVID-19 Diagnosis and Death.* Available at: https://www.gov.uk/government/publications/covid-19-pre-existing-health-conditions-and-ethnicity

Public Health England (PHE) (2021a) *Health Profile for England 2021.* Available at: https://fingertips.phe.org.uk/static-reports/health-profile-for-england/hpfe_report.html

Public Health England (PHE) (2021b) *Guidance: Health Visiting and School Nursing Service Delivery Model.* Available at: www.gov.uk/government/publications/commissioning-of-public-health-services-for-children/health-visiting-and-school-nursing-service-delivery-model#:~:text=Health%20visitors%20and%20school%20nurses%20provide%20continuity%20of%20care%20and,to%20other%20support%20and%20information.

Public Health England (PHE) (2022) *All Our Health: Personalised Care and Population Health.* Available at: https://www.gov.uk/government/collections/all-our-health-personalised-care-and-population-health

Public Services (Social Value) Act (2012). Available at: www.legislation.gov.uk/ukpga/2012/3/enacted

Purnell, L (2002) The Purnell Model of Cultural Competence. *Journal of Transcultural Nursing,* 13(3): 193–6.

Rayner, G and Lang, T (2012) *Ecological Public Health: Reshaping the Conditions for Good Health.* London: Routledge.

Razaq, A, Harrison, D, Karunanithi, S, Barr, B, Asaria, M, Routen, A and Khunti, K (2020) *BAME COVID-19 DEATHS – What Do We Know? Rapid Data and Evidence Review.* Available at: www.cebm.net/covid-19/bame-covid-19-deaths-what-do-we-know-rapid-data-evidence-review/ [Last Accessed: 13.09.22].

Rito, AI, Buoncristiano, M, Spinelli, A, Salanave, B, Kunešová, M and Hejgaard, T (2019) Association Between Characteristics at Birth, Breastfeeding and Obesity in 22 Countries: The WHO European Childhood Obesity Surveillance Initiative – COSI 2015/2017. *Obesity Facts,* 12: 226–43.

Ritzer, G, Dean, P and Jurgenson, N (2012) The Coming of Age of the Prosumer. *American Behavioural Scientist,* 56(4): 379–98.

Roberts, J and Bell, R (2015) *Social Inequalities in the Leading Causes of Early Death: A Life Course Approach.* Available at: www.instituteofhealthequity.org/resources-reports/social-inequalities-in-the-leading-causes-of-early-death-a-life-course-approach

Robertson, PJ, Roberts, DR and Porras, J (1993) Dynamics of Planned Organisational Change: Assessing Empirical Support for a Theoretical Model. *Academy of Management Journal,* 36(3): 619–35.

Robertson, R (2016) *Six Ways in Which NHS Financial Pressures Can Affect Patient Care.* Available at: www.kingsfund.org.uk/publications/six-ways

Rogers, EM (1983) *Diffusion of Innovations,* 3rd edition. New York: Macmillan.

Rosenstock, I (1974) Historical Origins of the Health Belief Model. *Health Education Monographs,* 2: 4.

Rouleau, G, Gagnon, MP and Côté, J (2015) Impacts of Information and Communication Technologies on Nursing Care: An Overview of Systematic Reviews (Protocol). *Systematic Reviews,* 4: 75.

Round, R, Marshall, B and Horton, K (2005) *Planning for Effective Health Promotion Evaluation.* Available at:

www.semanticscholar.org/paper/Planning-for-effective-health-promotion-evaluation-Round-Marshall/dcb282f1aaa32d724b15ca4c75b59ca4baebe269

Royal College of Nursing (RCN) (2017) *Healthy Workplace Toolkit for an Agency Workforce.* London: RCN.

Royal College of Nursing (RCN) (2019) *Healthy You.* Available at: www.rcn.org.uk/healthy-workplace/healthy-you

Royal Society for Public Health (RSPH) (2019) *Waking Up to the Health Benefits of Sleep.* Oxford: RSPH and Oxford University Press.

Royal Society for the Prevention of Accidents (ROSPA) (2018) *Road Safety Factsheet: Cycle Helmets.* London: ROSPA.

Saigal, S and Doyle, LW (2008) An Overview of Mortality and Sequelae of Preterm Birth from Infancy to Adulthood. *The Lancet,* 371(9608): 261–9.

Scottish Government (2015) *Scotland's Carers.* Available at: www.gov.scot/publications/scotlands-carers/pages/3/

Scriven, M (1991) *Evaluation Thesaurus,* 4th edition. Newbury Park, CA: SAGE.

Shelter (2018) *320,000 People in Britain Are Now Homeless, as Numbers Keep Rising.* Available at: https://england.shelter.org.uk/media/press_release/320,000_people_in_britain_are_now_homeless,_as_numbers_keep_rising

Sigerist, HE (1941) *Medicine and Human Welfare.* New Haven, CT: Yale University Press.

Simone, B, Carrillo-Santisteve, P and Lopalco, PL (2012) Healthcare Workers' Role in Keeping MMR Vaccination Uptake High in Europe: A Review of Evidence. *Eurosurveillance,* 17(26): 20206.

Skills for Care (2019) *Building Your Own Resilience, Health and Wellbeing.* Leeds: Skills for Care.

Social Care Institute for Excellence (SCIE) (2019) *Carers' Lives and Caring Issues: Knowledge and Research Evidence.* Available at: https://www.scie.org.uk/carers/knowledge-review/impact

Steel, N, Ford, JA, Newton, JN, Davis, ACJ, Vos, T and Naghavi, M (2018) Changes in Health in the Countries of the UK and 150 English Local Authority Areas 1990–2016: A Systematic Analysis for the Global Burden of Disease Study 2016. *The Lancet,* 392(10158): 1647–61.

Taber, JM, Leyva, B and Persoskie, A (2015) Why Do People Avoid Medical Care? A Qualitative Study Using National Data. *Journal of General Internal Medicine,* 30(3): 290–7.

Tanner, K and Allen, D (2007) Cultural competence in the College Biology Classroom. *CBE: Life Sciences Education,* 6(4): 251–8.

Tello, J and Barbazza, E (2015) *Health Services Delivery: A Concept Note.* WHO, Health Services Delivery Programme Regional Office for Europe. Available at: www.euro.who.int/__data/assets/pdf_file/0020/291611/Health-Services-Delivery-A-concept-note-301015.pdf

The Health Literacy Place (2022) *Toolkit: Techniques.* Available at: https://healthliteracyplace.org.uk/toolkit/techniques/

Thimbleby, H (2013) Technology and the Future of Healthcare. *Journal of Public Health Research*, 2(3): e28.

UK Government (2021) *The Green Book, Immunisation Against Infectious Diseases.* Available at: /www.gov.uk/government/collections/immunisation-against-infectious-disease-the-green-book

UK Government (2022) *Build Back Better: Our Plan for Health and Social Care.* Available at: www.gov.uk/government/publications/build-back-better-our-plan-for-health-and-social-care/build-back-better-our-plan-for-health-and-social-care

UK Health Security Agency (2019a) *Increasing Vaccine Uptake: Strategies for Addressing Barriers in Primary Care.* Available at: https://ukhsa.blog.gov.uk/2019/05/16/increasing-vaccine-uptake-strategies-for-addressing-barriers-in-primary-care/

UK Health Security Agency (2019b) *Measles in England.* Available at: https://ukhsa.blog.gov.uk/2019/08/19/measles-in-england/

UK Health Security Agency (UKHSA) (2022a) *Routine Childhood Immunisations from February 2022 (Born on or after 1 January 2020).* Available at: www.gov.uk/government/publications/routine-childhood-immunisation-schedule/routine-childhood-immunisations-from-february-2022-born-on-or-after-1-january-2020

UK Health Security Agency (UKHSA) (2022b) *Community-Centred and Asset-Based Approaches.* Available at: https://ukhsalibrary.koha-ptfs.co.uk/practice-examples/caba/

UK in a Changing Europe (2019) *Brexit and Public Opinion 2019.* Available at: https://ukandeu.ac.uk/wp-content/uploads/2019/01/Public-Opinion-2019-report.pdf

United Nations (UN) (2015) *Global Goals for Sustainable Development.* Available at: www.globalgoals.org

United Nations Children's Fund (UNICEF) (2019) *Baby Friendly Standards.* Available at: www.unicef.org.uk/babyfriendly/about/standards/

Welch, V, Petkovic, J, Pardo, JP, Rader, T and Tugwell, P (2016) Interactive Social Media Interventions to Promote Health Equity: An Overview of Reviews. *Health Promotion and Chronic Disease Prevention in Canada*, 36(4): 63–75.

Wenzel, L and Evans, H (2019) *Clicks and Mortar: Technology and the NHS Estate.* London: King's Fund.

Whitehead, D (2018) Exploring Health Promotion and Health Education in Nursing. *Nursing Standard*, 33(8): 38–44.

Wigan Council (2019) *The Deal.* Available at: www.wigan.gov.uk/Council/The-Deal/index.aspx

Willis, J (2022) *Foundations for Health Promotion*, 5th edition. London: Elsevier.

World Health Organization (WHO) (1985) *Targets for Health for All: Targets in Support of the European Strategy for Health for All.* Copenhagen: WHO Regional Office for Europe.

World Health Organization (WHO) (1986) *Ottawa Charter for Health Promotion.* Geneva: WHO.

World Health Organization (WHO) (1998) *Health Promotion Evaluation: Recommendations to Policy-Makers. Report of the WHO European Working Group on Health Promotion Evaluation.* Copenhagen: WHO Regional Office for Europe.

World Health Organization (WHO) (2001) *Evaluation in Health Promotion: Principles and Perspectives.* WHO Regional Publications, European Series, No. 92.

World Health Organization (WHO) (2006) *Working Together for Health: The World Health Report 2006.* Geneva: WHO.

World Health Organization (WHO) (2009) *Track 2: Health Literacy and Health Behaviour. 7th Global Conference on Health Promotion: Track Themes.* Available at: www.who.int/teams/health-promotion/enhanced-wellbeing/seventh-global-conference/health-literacy

World Health Organization (WHO) (2014) *Governance for Health Equity: Taking Forward the Equity Values and Goals of Health 2020 in the WHO European Region.* Geneva: WHO.

World Health Organization (WHO) (2016) *From Innovation to Implementation: eHealth in the WHO European Region.* Copenhagen: WHO Regional Office for Europe.

World Health Organization (WHO) (2017) *WHO Strategic Communications Framework for Effective Communications.* Geneva: WHO.

World Health Organization (WHO) (2019) *Health Impact Assessment (HIA).* Available at: www.who.int/tools/health-impact-assessments#:~:text=Health%20Impact%20Assessment%20%28HIA%29%20is%20a%20practical%20approach,a%20population%2C%20particularly%20on%20vulnerable%20or%20disadvantaged%20groups

World Health Organization (2020) *Measles and Rubella Strategic Framework 2021–2030.* Geneva: WHO. Available at: www.who.int/publications/i/item/measles-and-rubella-strategic-framework-2021-2030

Index